The Electronic Physician

DATE DUE

The Electronic Physician

GUIDELINES FOR IMPLEMENTING
A PAPERLESS PRACTICE

GOVERNORS STATE UNIVERSITY
UNIVERSITY PARK, IL

ALLSCRIPTS

ALLSCRIPTS™
Inform. Connect. Transform.

Chicago, IL

Published by Allscripts Healthcare Solutions
222 Merchandise Mart Plaza, Suite 2024
Chicago, IL 60654

Publisher's Cataloging-in-Publication Data
The electronic physician : guidelines for implementing a paperless practice / [edited by Todd Stein for Allscripts Healthcare Solutions]. —Chicago : Allscripts Healthcare Solutions, 2005.

p. ; cm.
Includes bibliographical references.
ISBN: 0-9765068-0-7

1. Medical records—Data processing. 2. Medical records—Management. 3. Information storage and retrieval systems—Medicine. I. Title. II. Stein, Todd. III. Allscripts Healthcare Solutions.

R864 .E44 2005
651.5/04261—dc22   2005-900631

Book production and coordination by
Jenkins Group, Inc. • www.bookpublishing.com
Interior design by Debbie Sidman
Cover design by Chris Rhoads

Printed in the United States of America
09 08 07 06 • 5 4 3

Contents

Acknowledgments

This book was authored by the following individuals:

Jed Batchelder	Maryse Laforce
Bruce Buerger	Laurie McGraw
Michael Cassarino	Dan Michelson
Jason Carmichael	Matt Nice
Simon Curtis	Bonnie Schirato
Peter Geerlofs, M.D.	Andrew Sears
Christina Godwin	Jerry Seufert
Brian Krupski	Glen Tullman

We'd like to express a special thank you to the following contributors:

The Abreon Group	John Jacksack
Maureen Augustin	Craig Luce
Scott Becker	Guy Mansueto
Melissa Bell	Steve Marth
Jim Bresee	David Nuckols
Karen Bunch	Mariann Olewnik
Liz Champagne	Sue Ordway
Doug Cobb	Paul Peterson
Mike Dow	Sue Simmons
Erin Ennis	Eileen Waters
Karl Greiter	Linda Winslow
Jill Helm	Matt Woodside
Killian Hermann	

Additionally, we'd like to acknowledge the efforts of our editor, Todd Stein.

Most importantly we would like to extend our thanks to over 1,500 clinics across the United States who have implemented Electronic Health Record solutions from Allscripts!

Introduction

Nearly three decades have elapsed since the Electronic Medical Record (EMR) was first conceived, and more than 15 years have passed since the Institute of Medicine's first report called for the implementation of computerized patient records. And yet, from day one, there was never a doubt that an EMR could dramatically improve patient care, reduce errors, save physician time and remove significant cost and duplication from the healthcare system. In fact, on more than one occasion, respected individuals have claimed that the EHR could have as powerful an impact on patient care as the discovery of penicillin.

Unfortunately, the reality of EMRs hasn't kept pace with the promise. Despite hundreds of millions of dollars invested, the EMR largely failed, until recently, to win over physicians and therefore had minimal impact on patient care. Why would such a promising technology go virtually unused for so long? The answer brings to light some of the key challenges facing today's complex healthcare system.

First Generation Mistakes

The first generation of EMRs were "sold to CIOs and told to physicians"—a phrase that expresses the lack of widespread physician involvement and buy-in. The result of this approach was predictably sub-optimal, at best. The rare physicians who became involved in the EMR process were generally professionals with a deep interest in clinical technology who had long been convinced of its benefits. These high-profile innovators, early adopters and committed change agents were mostly to be found at academic medical centers, which had the resources to overcome the inconvenience and extra work associated with the early EMRs.

By contrast, the average physician struggling under a heavy workload at a busy multi-specialty practice just couldn't afford the hassle and the expense of adopting an EMR. The problem was that EMRs simply were not mainstream enough to appeal to most healthcare organizations, and few people were willing to acknowledge this truth, especially given the amount of money spent and the high-profile individuals associated with the early EMR programs. The Emperor's Clothes phenomenon prevented anyone from telling key administrators and physicians that the technology actually didn't work, so real progress was delayed.

During this period—call it the last ten years—healthcare costs continued to escalate and quality problems continued to multiply at an unacceptable rate. The system was not only broken, it was headed for a crash landing. The sheer enormity of the problem forced stakeholders across the healthcare environment to take notice, and the sleeping giant awoke at last. General Motors complained that it was spending more on healthcare than it did on steel for its cars, and a chorus of employers from every industry voiced fears that rising healthcare costs would hurt their ability to compete.

Around the same time, the Institute of Medicine published a high-profile report estimating that nearly 100,000 Americans died unnecessarily each year as a result of preventable medical errors. The report made front-page news across the nation and the globe. Meanwhile, the rising number of people without health insurance highlighted an intractable problem that began to spur politicians to action. And, last but surely not least, consumers, who in healthcare are called patients, became impatient with the lack of available information. They were becoming accustomed to using the Internet to handle virtually every other kind of transaction and they wanted the same benefits and information from healthcare. At the same time, consumers (and healthcare organizations) realized that much of the expense in healthcare was preventable or manageable with better information. Given this set of demands, the EMR began to morph into an Electronic Health Record or EHR, which included patient access, input, portability and connectivity to their health records. In acknowledgement of this broadening scope, we have used the term EHR throughout this book because in the new age of healthcare, an EMR is just a subset of what's needed to succeed.

EHRs Cross the Chasm

Recently, the energy behind automating healthcare and raising it to the technological level of every other major industry has been substantial. The market has reached the moment that Andy Grove, the former CEO of Intel, called an "inflection point" or, to use the latest terminology, the "Tipping Point." Between 2003 and 2004, the number of healthcare professionals converted to the benefits of automation rose so quickly that the group tipped from innovators and early adopters to what Geoffrey Moore, in his book "Crossing the Chasm," called the "early majority."

Once dismissed as a technologist's pipe dream, the EHR today is being embraced by every healthcare organization. The question is no longer "should we purchase an EHR," but rather, "which one should we buy and how quickly can we deploy it?" No respected CEO, CIO or CMO would dismiss the need for EHRs, any more than they would dismiss the need for quality. Indeed, market forces are increasingly making EHRs *the* standard of care.

Recent breakthroughs in technology and deployment have also contributed to the adoption of EHRs. These changes include the arrival of lower cost, higher quality mobile, wireless technologies such as notebook computers, Tablet PCs and PDAs. As more and more physicians began using these technologies outside of their practice, physician-centered software that was easy to learn and use also began to be more available. At the same time, there was a growing understanding that physician adoption is a change management process. Each of these factors contributed to the rapid acceleration of EHR usage.

Keeping the Focus on Physicians

At Allscripts, our vision from the beginning has been all about physicians and becoming an indispensable part of the way physicians practice medicine. Physicians are front and center in our universe. One of our physicians coined the phrase, "If Doctors Don't Use It, Nothing Else Matters," referred to throughout this book by the acronym IDDUINEM. To embrace this philosophy is not to say that others in the process are unimportant. Executive sponsorship is critical to a successful implementation, as is the support of nurses, other caregivers and administrative staff. But to achieve all the benefits of an EHR, nothing is more important than having the physicians on board, leading the way and making the technology and software a part of their routine.

Today, the question is no longer whether an EHR can deliver benefits (that's been established) or whether you need one, or even *when* you need one—because the EHR has arrived. The real question is, how do you deploy an EHR and realize its benefits?

That's what this book is about. Our goal was to create a useful guide for those who are currently deploying an electronic health record or about to deploy one.

It's important to note that this is not a promotional exercise. The book is an outgrowth of Allscripts' Six Sigma efforts to put into place a standardized process for our own deployments, and to share knowledge with our team and clients.

And as we all know, standardization and best practices lead to higher quality and reduced costs. While the contributors to the book are all employees or clients of Allscripts, our aim was to produce an objective guide and overview of the entire EHR implementation process—a guide that would be helpful to any reader, regardless of which vendor they choose. That said, we believe Allscripts is in a unique position to deliver first-hand observations and advice from which everyone can benefit. The authors drew on real life lessons (some more painful than others) and analysis of more than 140 organizations representing in excess of 1,500 individual clinics that have implemented Allscripts' EHR solutions over the last two years, along with original research and other published sources.

With a target audience of physicians, practice executives, managers, and project managers, the book covers a wide range of topics, including guidelines for forming effective project teams, basic technology requirements, change management, advice for improving physician adoption, and ROI planning, measurement and analysis.

Some readers may feel that a software company like Allscripts should stick to software, but they would be missing the point: An electronic health record implementation is not about the software. World-class software paired with a commitment from your vendor to work side-by-side with your organization is critical, but it's not enough. Success depends upon putting in place the right leadership structures, the right processes, and the right kind of change management. That, and the unshakeable conviction of the organization that, no matter what, there is no turning back—a message best delivered by the Chief Executive and the most senior physician leader.

Underneath it all lays the simple process of learning. We have a philosophy at Allscripts that may help, more than anything, to explain this book:

What we don't know, we teach each other.

With thanks to our clients, from whom we have learned and together with whom we continue to learn every day, we present our best ideas, experiences, reflections and creative solutions for making your EHR a success. We hope and trust that you will find our observations useful on the road ahead. Healthcare and countless patients are depending on us to figure this out.

Glen Tullman
Chief Executive Officer, Allscripts
January 2005

Foreword

The Electronic Physician: MIT's Journey from Vision to Reality

By Tom Goodwin, MHA, Director of Clinical Information Systems, Massachusetts Institute of Technology Medical

In the late 1990's, the Medical Department at the Massachusetts Institute of Technology began a lengthy journey to implement an electronic medical record (EMR). At the time, we were little more than pioneers walking a poorly marked trail with a crude compass. Like the rest of the healthcare industry, we weren't quite sure how to get from the EMR vision to reality. But we were sustained by the hopeful notion that things would be better when we reached our goal—an electronic scheduling system, a standardized billing system, a reporting tool and, if we were lucky, something that would replicate the paper record without intruding on our clinicians.

From the beginning, we moved forward, though not necessarily in a straight line or at a consistent pace. Our travel through the unexplored territory was often hostile and uncertain but we caused no mass uprising and, thanks eventually to the implementation of the TouchWorks EMR from Allscripts, we managed to achieve breakthrough results that we believe improved the quality of care we provide while saving us time and money. As a result of our efforts, and the efforts of countless other organizations, the journey to an EHR is now along a worn but sure path. The destination is well worth the effort it takes to get there, and this book can help serve as your guide.

At MIT Medical, we began our journey in 1998 with an exhaustive search for a Clinical Information System (CIS). Our Steering Committee chose IDX Systems Corp., based on its strength in practice management. As a bonus, IDX tossed in an early version of an electronic medical record known as the Clinical Management System (CMS).

The clinical side at MIT Medical had a simple first goal. We wanted to make laboratory results available via computer before the much-feared (and over-hyped) Y2K bug rendered our laboratory computer system obsolete. We beat the millennium's arrival by a month and a half and were able to back-fill a year's worth of laboratory results along with patient demographic information and clinician schedules. Lab results were then fed continuously in real time into the CIS. To provide comfort to our clinicians, paper laboratory reports were still printed twice daily and hand delivered to the various clinician offices in our building.

Meanwhile, MIT Medical Department's conversion from a rag-tag paper appointment system to the IDX scheduling system took place throughout 1999. Early on we made what appeared to be a near fatal decision to decentralize patient appointment booking. The change was too ambitious, and we lacked the critical ingredient of buy-in from clinicians, as well as the firm support of the administration. Suddenly, with no real transition, we abandoned our previously small, dedicated scheduling staff and instructed patients to call the clinician's cluster to make their appointments. Secretaries instantly became appointment makers because we assumed they would know the patient and clinician better than anyone. We hired outside resources to train the secretaries but the training happened too far in advance of implementation and it was not customized sufficiently to our environment. As a result, our secretaries were spending lots of extra time on the phone handling appointments and they were less available to clinicians and patients with non-scheduling questions.

The department's struggle with adapting the scheduling software to our environment was nearly crippling. Frustration and anger put tremendous pressure on the Project Team to perfect the rollout of the upcoming IDX billing system and further clinical functionality. Meanwhile, MIT Medical's clinicians were becoming concerned that the clinical system would get in the way of their medical practice. The clinicians had no interest in doing clerical work and they worried that patients would be suspicious of online access to their personal medical information. But many clinicians liked the idea of having near-instant lab results available without having to call the laboratory or wait several days for the paper reports to be delivered.

During the summer of 2000, while work was continuing on the IDX billing system, the Project Team met to discuss feeding transcriptions into our clinical system. We spent an excessive amount of time getting consensus on the font for the paper reports. We were not bold when thinking about transcription and didn't immediately see how important it was to have an accurate note as the central element of the clinical system. We expected to continue to print paper transcriptions, have clinicians edit and sign the papers, and then file them into the paper record. The electronic feed into the clinical system was intended only as a repository of unedited, unsigned notes.

When the IDX billing system finally went live in June 2001, we added a five-year history of radiology reports to the system along with a real-time interface for new radiology reports. In March 2002 we began populating our clinical system with all of the filled prescriptions from our in-house pharmacy. This was the crude start to an electronic patient medication list. By early 2002 we were ready to continue our journey with the crude beginnings of an electronic patient medication list as we began populating our clinical system with filled prescriptions from our in-house pharmacy.

We had always known that the core function of a clinical information system is its ability to retrieve clinical data. But we failed to foresee how a CIS could improve workflow and organizational efficiency. Instead, we devoted ourselves to merely replicating the existing paper record. It was a failure of vision that we attempted to correct with our first real venture into paradigm change in the summer of 2002. That's when we began using the CIS to track patient-clinician phone calls. This was the first time our clinicians documented interactions electronically. Instantly, a second volume of the patient record was born.

The next challenge was getting clinicians to *use* the CIS for documentation. This required that we find an individual clinician—preferably one of some standing—to act as the new system's champion and to assist in nailing down a workflow those other clinicians would accept. In our case, we relied on Dr. David Shein, whose willingness to develop functional workflows for the new system was invaluable.

Another key ingredient to success was having support from senior clinician leadership. Our Medical Director, William Kettyle, mandated the use of our CIS for documenting patient-clinician phone interactions. This was a giant step forward in an organization that has traditionally shied away from mandates. But we took this drastic step because we were convinced that no system, whether electronic, paper, or hybrid, would work if its use was optional and not standardized. Astonishingly, all clinicians went along with the mandate and there was very little grumbling.

During the fall of 2002 clinicians began electronically verifying laboratory and radiology results online. At that time, laboratory and radiology reports stopped being filed in the paper chart. Laboratory reports were still printed and distributed as a safety net but they were shredded without being placed in the paper chart. This furthered our commitment to the electronic medical record.

In March of 2003 we upgraded the client server (visual basic Clinical Management System) to the Web-based TouchWorks system from Allscripts, which integrates seamlessly with IDX's information systems. We took that opportunity to institute mandatory electronic editing and signature of clinical notes in TouchWorks without printing for the paper chart. Initially, our transcription costs increased but we gained efficiency by avoiding printing and saved money by reducing the need for filing thousands of paper reports. Eventually, we changed transcription vendors and used more direct note entry. As a result, our transcription expenditures have since dropped significantly.

At the same time, we also began offering clinicians secure remote access to our clinical information. They were now able to access patient's medical records while they were making rounds at local hospitals or even from their homes. In July 2003, with the completion of an electronic interface from the TouchWorks system to our in-house pharmacy, we began offering electronic prescribing. This helped increase patient safety, reduced phone calls, and made our pharmacy staff more efficient. We also were able to redesign our medication renewal workflow, allowing clinicians to fill patient requests with a few simple clicks.

Impressed by the early results from TouchWorks, in October 2003 we purchased Allscripts' Scan application. When we went live with Scan, we stopped filing outside consults, as well as any other documents that would previously have been filed into the paper record. Instead, a scanned image of the document was available instantly at the clinician's fingertips. Additionally, in June 2004 we implemented a TouchWorks' orders interface that allows clinicians to order and track lab tests.

There is no doubt the EHR has helped us manage patient care more efficiently and cost-effectively. Once an organization gets past replicating the paper record and experiences the EHR's potential for improving workflows, there is a true opportunity to transform and dramatically improve the practice, both on the business side and in the clinic. With perseverance, innovation, and the help and guidance of Allscripts, we at MIT Medical were able to accomplish far better results than we dreamed possible.

Editor's Note

The electronic health record suffers from a rare disease called acronym confusion. Although it has been adopted by thousands of health care institutions across the globe, we're still not exactly sure what to call it. Over time, at least three different acronyms have taken hold: CPR (computer-based patient record), EMR (electronic medical record) and, most recently, EHR (electronic health record).

Unfortunately, each of these terms carries a different meaning. Generally speaking, CPR is used to describe an electronic record that combines information from both ambulatory and hospital settings. EMR is usually meant to connote an ambulatory tool that's for doctors only and something that replaces the paper record with a database. Finally, EHR was coined to describe a fully evolved electronic record system— one that not only includes the patient but also may be used by the patient, and which also provides a set of tools that improve workflow efficiency and quality of care in doctors' offices.

For simplicity's sake—and because we believe it's the most accurate term—we have used EHR throughout this book to describe any digital medical record, except in discussions of the technology's evolution from the earlier EMR.

CHAPTER ONE

Driving Forces:
A Brief History of the EHR

In This Chapter
- Why the EHR is the new stethoscope
- Early challenges to EHR acceptance
- The impact of medical errors
- EHRs cross the chasm

Since the dawn of the computer era, few new ideas have so intrigued physicians as the electronic medical record, or EMR. When it was introduced in the 1970s, the EMR promised major improvements upon the old paper record: freedom from paperwork, greater speed, remote access, improved patient safety, lower costs, even enhanced reimbursements. But until recently, very few physicians actually used an EMR in their practices. The technology was cumbersome, time consuming and expensive, and most physicians were unwilling to take a chance on a technology that hadn't been widely adopted by their peers.

Today, it's a different story. More than 30 percent of mid- to large-size practices either already use or are in the process of implementing an Electronic Health Record (EHR)—an expanded version of the earlier EMR. The EHR is quickly becoming a standard part of the way care is delivered in the U.S. What changed? As we'll discuss in this chapter, the EHR's mainstreaming is the story of a "perfect storm"—a combination of technological advances and powerful societal changes that forced the hand of employers and large payers, energized legislators, empowered patients and awakened physicians to the promise of computerized medicine.

The New Stethoscope

An interesting historical analogy to the slow but gradual rate of EHR adoption can be found in the introduction of the simple stethoscope. In 1834, when stethoscopes were first sold, *The London Times* ran this unflattering review of the new technology: "That it will ever come into general use, notwithstanding its value, is extremely doubtful because its beneficial application requires much time and gives a good bit of trouble, both to the patient and to the practitioner because its hue and character are foreign and opposed to all our habits and associations."

Eventually, of course, the stethoscope became commonplace—today, most physicians couldn't imagine practicing medicine without one. Yet its widespread adoption didn't happen overnight. Like all new technologies, the stethoscope experienced a sudden, massive increase in adoption only after it reached the stage (referred to in the Introduction) called the "tipping point." This is the sudden turning point found in the life cycle of every successful product or idea where seemingly overnight, it becomes ubiquitous. At the beginning of the product life cycle, a small number of innovators and early adopters are quick to see the value in the new technology.

Today, the EHR has reached its tipping point and is quickly becoming a standard part of the way healthcare is delivered in the U.S. Before we detail the technology's future, it's important to look back at mistakes that were made on the EHR's path to acceptance that contributed to its slow adoption rate. As the saying goes, if we don't learn from the past, we're destined to repeat it.

Early Challenges in EHR Acceptance

While many have blamed the initially slow adoption rate of EHRs on problems with the technology, or physicians' resistance to change, we believe the real cause lies elsewhere, in four key failures. Because many organizations continue to repeat the same mistakes, it's critical that we understand these early failures and learn from them. The first serious shortcoming of the early EHRs was their all-or-nothing, monolithic approach to implementation, which unfortunately often meant nothing was done. Since the early EHRs could not be implemented one function or module at a time (e.g., prescribing, then charge capture, then document management and retrieval, etc.), physicians almost universally rejected a wholesale change in their practice patterns as too much, too soon, and too risky.

A second shortcoming of early EHRs was that they were neither user friendly or intuitive enough to be used in a productive fashion. They tried to completely change the physician's workflow and took more, not less, time. In addition, there was typically not enough training or support for physicians who were expected to embrace new technology and a changed workflow, often without changing their patient loads.

A third shortcoming of the early EHRs was that they were not comprehensive. The early systems often fell short of providing full functionality by automating only some of what physicians did and providing little of the information they needed to access. They typically offered no pathway for a complete record or complete automation and very little connectivity.

Which leads to the final shortcoming. Early EHRs were stand-alone applications that did not fully integrate with existing in-house systems (such as practice management) or link with outside systems (laboratories and hospitals). They were islands in a sea of information. If physicians had to handle some paper and regularly go outside the system, they saw no benefit to partial automation. In fact, physicians regularly printed out the file from the EHR and had it filed with the paper record, so all the information would be together.

Despite the obvious shortcomings of the early EHRs, vendors and other proponents regularly blamed physicians for failing to use the applications, calling them "technology averse." When you consider that physicians were among the first professionals in any industry to adopt pagers and cell phones and that they frequently use cutting-edge and complex diagnostic and surgical equipment, it's clear that the technology-phobic label was neither fair nor accurate.

In fact, physicians have consistently proved that they will use a new technology that provides a real return on effort (ROE)—they make an instant assessment if something is actually worth their time. For a long time, EHRs failed to deliver reasonable ROE. While their relatively high cost was considered at the time to be the primary obstacle to adoption, the real challenge was time: early EHR's actually took more time and to this day, many of the benefits of the basic automation that an EHR provides accrue to other stakeholders in the healthcare system. How could physicians be expected to rapidly adopt a technology that hadn't yet proven itself worthwhile to them?

What Silver Bullet?

For years, healthcare IT experts had been predicting a market-transforming event that would launch the widespread adoption of EHRs. But the silver bullet never arrived. Instead, the turning point for EHR adoption was driven by an unexpected combination of economic requirements, technological advances and powerful social changes. The most visible part of the process began in 1999, when the Institute of Medicine (IOM)—Congress's lead advisory group on healthcare issues—reported that preventable medical errors kill 98,000 Americans every year. The IOM's report made headlines across the country and marked the beginning of an acute awareness among the general public and healthcare insiders that the healthcare system was fundamentally broken.

However, underlying the quality concerns was an economic issue that business had been struggling with for years: the cost of healthcare. Employers used the release of the IOM report and the resulting public pressure to reduce the number of deaths from medical errors to spur a number of private and public initiatives. One of the most visible efforts was the Leapfrog Group, a high-profile coalition of 150 of the nation's largest employers, who pay a high price for employee health benefits and yet have little control over the cost and quality of the care their employees receive. To help the public understand the costs, General Motors reported that for every car it produced, it spent more on healthcare benefits than on steel.

Leapfrog began pressuring hospitals to adopt a patient safety plan that included Computerized Physician Order Entry (CPOE). As Leapfrog built pressure to address patient safety via clinical automation, two things became crystal clear: first, that healthcare providers didn't have access to the information they needed to understand, target and improve their processes; and, second, that the high cost of healthcare could largely be attributed to the effort to identify key disease states, proactively manage them, and treat patients outside the four walls of the hospital. By the time the patient was in the hospital, it was too late to provide cost-effective care. These realizations triggered a number of significant efforts that focused on technology adoption, the standards needed to facilitate a more connected healthcare system, better patient access to information, and pay-for-performance programs. Some of the more visible efforts included the e-healthcare initiative, the Markel Foundation and the HL7 standards task force.

More and more studies began to support this notion of healthcare delivery outside the hospital. According to the National Center for Health Statistics, more than half of all healthcare is now delivered in physician's offices, for a staggering total of more than 1 billion patient visits per year. Moreover, a rash of studies suggest that medical errors are not only more widespread than the IOM numbers suggest, but that they are deeply rooted in the ambulatory setting:

- A July 2004 study by Health Grades, Inc. found that the number of annual deaths from medical errors is nearly 195,000—double the IOM's estimate. "If the Center for Disease Control's annual list of leading causes of death included medical errors, it would show up as number six, ahead of diabetes, pneumonia, Alzheimer's disease and renal disease," said Samantha Collier, MD, vice president of medical affairs at Health Grades.

- A study by the Robert Graham Center in Washington, D.C. concluded that more patients are harmed by medical errors from care received in physicians' offices than in hospitals. The research, published in the April 2004 edition of the peer-reviewed journal Quality and Safety in Health Care, reviewed 5,921 malpractice claims that could be identified as errors. Of the errors found in the claims, 68 percent were negligent events in outpatient settings that resulted in more than 1,200 deaths.

- An earlier study by the Center for Information Technology Leadership (CITL) projected that the U.S. could save $44 billion annually by installing ambulatory computerized physician order entry (ACPOE) systems in every doctor's office. The savings would come from the nationwide system's ability to prevent more than 2 million adverse drug events, of which up to 130,000 are life threatening, the study found.

These and other prominent studies sparked significant attention at the federal level. Bipartisan support quickly developed for computerizing patient records in both the acute and ambulatory settings. Political pundits joked that healthcare IT was the only issue that could unite President George W. Bush, Senator John Kerry, Senator Hillary Rodham Clinton, Newt Gingrich and Senator Ted Kennedy. This broad consensus quickly resulted in action. In early 2004, President Bush appointed David J. Brailer, MD, as National Health Information Technology Coordinator, a newly created position reporting to the Health and Human Services Secretary, to coordinate and accelerate the adoption of clinical information technology.

Within 90 days, Dr. Brailer introduced a plan outlining four goals:

1. Bring EHRs into clinical practice: Encourage incentives for EHR adoption, shared investments for technology, and support of electronic

records in clinical settings. Reduce the risks of changing clinical practice and operations with low-cost support systems. Improve adoption among providers in rural and underserved areas by encouraging technology transfer and other support.

2. Connect clinicians: Create health data exchange collaborations on the local level to connect health care workers and support the exchange of information for clinical decisions and treatments. Coordinate federal health systems to improve care, reimbursement procedures and oversight. As part of a national infrastructure, encourage development of a set of tools such as mobile authentication, Web architecture and security features.

3. Create more consumer-focused care: To help personalize care, encourage the widespread use of personal health records, greater ability for patients to choose providers based on factors such as care quality and an expansion of telemedicine services to reach patients in rural and underserved areas.

4. Improve population-based health: Integrate public health surveillance systems into an interoperable network that supports data exchange. . Encourage a similar infrastructure that brings together state and local data collection efforts, along with better information tools, to accelerate research and dissemination of results on care quality and other health issues.

As these goals were announced, Mark McClellan, the administrator for the Centers for Medicare and Medicaid Services (CMS), the organization ultimately responsible for approximately 30 percent of healthcare spending in this country, made the adoption of EHR/eRx technology a top priority and announced his intention to beat the 2009 deadline for adoption of standards for writing and transmitting electronic prescriptions.

Meanwhile, as the federal government moved to encourage healthcare information technology, a number of fundamental and important changes were occurring in the marketplace that further sped the EHR's transition into the mainstream.

Physicians Embrace the Computer

By the late '90s, computer applications were fast becoming a part of physicians' everyday lives both inside and outside the office. Although physicians continued to let their office staff handle the computerized billing and scheduling systems used in nearly every medical group, they quickly became adept at using e-mail and the Internet for their own purposes. These applications, it turned out, were the perfect introduction to computers because they were easy to use and delivered instant value. Soon, many physicians began to wonder why their 6-year-olds were using computers in school while they continued to rely on outdated paper systems for tracking patient care in the clinic.

Gradually, the average physicians' resistance to computerized medicine was displaced by curiosity about how computers could help make their practices more efficient and profitable. Additionally, physicians leaving residency had come to expect that computers would be a standard of care delivery when they entered private practice. Physicians' groups found it increasingly difficult to attract new physicians without having an EHR in place or at least a plan for implementing one.

One revealing anecdote on the emerging movement of EHRs into the mainstream came from the Chief Information Officer (CIO) of a large, prestigious, East Coast academic medical group. "Ask any CIO about their organization's EHR-implementation strategy," he said, "and if they haven't already deployed one, they're generally too embarrassed to admit it." In short, the question CIOs are asking themselves now is not if they should implement an EHR but when."

Recent studies support this conclusion. A 2003 survey of 464 medical groups by the Medical Group Management Association (MGMA), the largest association of medical groups in the nation, revealed that 62 percent of them planned to purchase an EHR in the next 24 months. And, a 2004 survey of 2400 medical groups (of seven or more physicians) conducted by Allscripts found that 33 percent had already purchased an EHR.

The Web Empowers Patients

While physicians and healthcare groups were fast embracing computerized medicine, another catalyst was busy transforming the traditional role of patients (and therefore physicians). Popular new web browsers like Netscape and Internet Explorer were beginning to draw millions of people to the Web for information of all kinds. Soon, literally hundreds of health-related websites were available at the touch of a mouse. Easy access to health information and scientific research that had previously been unavailable to most people began to transform the average passive patient into a well-informed, proactive healthcare consumer. Suddenly patients were arriving in their physician's office armed with information, and ready for discussion. Physicians found themselves taking on a new role. No longer the gatekeepers of medical information, they had to adjust to being interpreters and facilitators of vast stores of medical knowledge ubiquitously available to their patients. Their need for accurate and real-time access to information became ever more acute.

At the time, physicians who were still on the fence about EHRs received a push from the technology itself. Vendors began to unveil applications that were more secure, stable, and accessible. Another boost: the introduction of the 802.11 standard for wireless local area technology (WLAN) coupled with Web-based applications that for the first time enabled physicians to take the clinical record with them wherever they went.

It's hard to overestimate the importance of the wireless and web-based EHR to physicians' peace of mind. While other professionals routinely leave work at a reasonable hour, spend time with their families and then log on to their home computer to finish up loose ends at work, large numbers of physicians end their workday as late as 9 p.m. after struggling through a stack of patient charts and a jumble of sticky notes. The wireless and Web-based EHR has changed all that, allowing physicians to finish up their paperwork from the comfort of their own homes.

But mobility is not the only advantage physicians have gained from the EHR. To appreciate how the EHR has changed their lives, imagine going through every workday without knowing whom you'd be seeing in your next meeting or appointment. You would be unprepared for most meetings and more than a little anxious about the agenda and potential outcome. Unlikely, you say? Not so. Paperbound physicians face this untenable situation every day. With a paper schedule they might have a vague sense of the day's events but once things get rolling and walk-ins and cancellations happen, their schedule spins out of control. Something as simple as providing a real-time digital schedule is vital to physicians. It lets them know whether the next patient has arrived and, retrospectively, whether a note and a charge have been completed for each patient they saw that day. It's a quantum leap in terms of organization.

Physicians also lack control over another essential element of their workday—their clinical notes. Unlike other professionals, who can take their notes with them wherever they go and organize them in any way they choose, physicians are forced to hand over control of their notes to others. While they can create their notes in multiple ways (dictation, handwriting, etc.), they must then hand them off to a transcriptionist for entry into the record. After their notes are typed into the chart, they have to share the chart with other providers in their practice, thus losing control over how their notes (the chart) are organized and distributed. Then, when they need the chart, they're forced to wait until their request is routed through others. Finally, when they leave the clinic they no longer have access to the chart, even though patients will continue to require their help.

By contrast, an electronic chart compiles information from all sources (dictation, structured entry, scanned documents), presents the data in a consistent, organized and customizable manner, and is accessible anywhere at anytime.

Evidence of Financial Returns

The final ingredient that assured the mainstreaming of the EHR is the growing body of evidence that the applications can generate a positive financial return. One of the most compelling of these studies was published in the Winter 2004 issue of the *Journal of Healthcare Information Management*, the quarterly peer-reviewed publication of the Healthcare Information and Management Systems Society (HIMSS). The study, "The Economic Effect of Implementing an EMR in an Outpatient Clinical Setting," was conducted by Central Utah Clinic (CUC), the largest independent multi-specialty group in the state of Utah with (at the time) 59 physicians, nine locations and 200,000 active patients.

During the one-year period of the study, CUC experienced direct, measurable reductions in spending and increases in revenue from its Allscripts' TouchWorks EHR of more than $952,000 compared to the previous year, or approximately $20,000 per physician. This was the highest level of first-year savings ever documented in a peer-reviewed journal. The study's authors projected cumulative savings of more than $8.2 million over a five-year period. Savings were achieved due to reduced expenditures or increased revenue in the following areas:

- Reduced transcription costs
- Reductions in staff required for pulling, filing and maintaining charts
- Elimination of the cost of building charts for new patients
- Decreased physical space requirements due to a paperless record

- Increased revenue due to improved documentation and more appropriate reimbursement coding levels.

The authors concluded: "Taken together, these data confirm our findings that financial benefits will accrue to healthcare institutions from the implementation of an EMR. Moreover, the benefits may accrue more quickly, as in the case of CUC, than most past studies have projected."

Crossing the Chasm

We have described a number of powerful social and technological changes that contributed to moving the EHR into the mainstream of clinical practice: Society's urgent need to address medical errors, improve patient safety and deliver healthcare more cost effectively; the introduction of modular applications that let organizations deploy an EHR efficiently at their own pace; physicians' developing comfort level with clinical technology; the accumulation of data supporting ROI; the growing interest of patients in electronic records; and advances in wireless and web-based technology. Taken together, all of these forces have contributed to marketplace momentum.

Once dismissed as another promising new technology that would never take hold, the EHR is fast becoming a success story. After decades of market development, it has emerged as a new standard in the delivery of safe, efficient, cost-effective and high-quality patient care.

The Recap

- The EHR has reached its tipping point and is quickly becoming a standard part of the way healthcare is delivered in the U.S.

- A serious shortcoming of the first EMRs was their all-or-nothing approach to implementation, which unfortunately often meant nothing was done.

- The early systems often fell short of providing full functionality by offering incomplete or confusing workflows and no pathway for a complete record.

- Given the shortcomings of first generation EMRs, it was unfair of early proponents to label reluctant physicians "technology averse" for failing to use the applications.

- A 1998 Institute of Medicine (IOM) report that estimated 98,000 Americans die each year from preventable medical errors marked the beginning of an acute awareness among healthcare insiders and the general public that the healthcare system was a problem in need of a solution.

- The IOM report energized economic forces to begin to drive the EHR revolution.

- The appointment of David J. Brailer, M.D., Ph.D., as National Health Information Technology Coordinator, a newly created position reporting to the Health and Human Services Secretary, helped accelerate the adoption of clinical information technology.

- Gradually, the average physicians' distrust of computerized medicine was displaced by curiosity about how computers could help make their practices more efficient and profitable.

- The availability of consumer health information on the Internet transitioned the role of physicians from gatekeepers of medical information to being interpreters and facilitators of vast stores of medical knowledge ubiquitously available to their patients.

- The introduction of the 802.11 standard for wireless local area technology (WLAN), coupled with Web-based applications, enabled physicians for the first time to take the clinical record with them wherever they went.

- The final ingredient that assured the mainstreaming of the EHR is the growing body of evidence that the applications can generate a positive financial return on investment.

If You Have Time

- Toward an Electronic Patient Record '95: Eleventh International Symposium on the Creation of Electronic Health Records. C. Peter Waegemann, editor. Medical Records Institute. (March 1995).

- Essentials of Health Information Management: Principles and Practices. Michelle A. Green, Mary Jo Bowie. Thomson Delmar Learning. (August 2004).

- Health IT Strategic Framework. Office of the National Coordinator for Health Information Technology. (July 2004).

CHAPTER TWO

The EHR Mental Model: The Big Picture

IN THIS CHAPTER
- What makes it an EHR?
- Critical Attributes
- Core functions
- Decision support
- Reaching beyond the four walls

The EHR Mental Model

A mental model or conceptual framework is a vital prerequisite to operating any technology. You would not be able to use this book unless you possessed a mental model telling you how books work. Though you probably don't think of it as such, your mental model of this book includes the knowledge that flipping pages is the way to move through the text, and that you can access topical information by referring to the index. If it takes a working mental model to navigate a book, imagine trying to operate a system as complex as an electronic health record without one.

The first exhaustive definition of the Electronic Medical Record was developed in the early 1990s by Richard Dick, Elaine B. Steen and Don Detmer, authors of the landmark book, "The Computer-Based Patient Record: An Essential Technology for Healthcare." Building on their work, the EHR mental model presented here has two goals: First, to stretch your understanding of what the EHR is and what it can accomplish for your patients and your practice; second, to provide a framework for understanding and even predicting how the EHR field will evolve over the next few years. The latter point is critical because we expect the capabilities of the EHR to change dramatically in coming years as more physicians begin to use information systems and demand more sophisticated capabilities. If you can predict roughly how the current systems will evolve, you'll be able to choose the best EHR for your current and future needs.

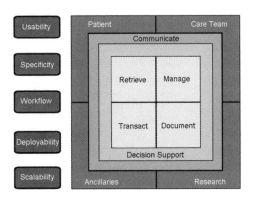

The EHR Mental Model

The EHR Mental Model we'll discuss in this chapter includes the main attributes and functional components of an electronic health record. In the diagram above you can see a list of general attributes on the left that are critical to the success of an EHR. On the right is a representation of an EHR's functional components and how they interact with one another and the user. Notice that the core functions—retrieve, manage, transact and document—are at the center of the diagram while the outer squares represent more advanced functionalities that operate within and beyond the four walls of the physicians' office.

We'll begin our discussion with the five EHR attributes that are key to success in today's healthcare marketplace.

Critical Attributes of the EHR

Usability

Obviously, the most critical element of any EHR is its usability. If your clinicians refuse to use the new EHR, you can forget all about improved quality and efficiency, reduced costs and a solid return on investment. To deliver these benefits, an EHR must first provide a positive user experience, which in turn requires an intuitive learning process, easy-to-retain directions, and flexibility in accommodating a variety of pathways to performing tasks.

Other chapters of this book will cover the many factors that influence physician utilization of an EHR, so we won't go into much detail on that subject here. But it's worth noting that one of the most important determinants of usability is ease of use. For years, it was mistakenly believed that physicians were slow to adopt EHRs because they were unfamiliar with computers and resisted using them in their practices. Whether that's true or not—and there's good reason to doubt the "computer-phobic" label—the bigger problem with early EHRs was their failure to satisfy physicians' everyday needs. Until recently, EHRs were simply too cumbersome and difficult to use, discouraging even the most highly motivated physicians. Faced with an expensive technology that satisfied few of their real needs, doctors complained, "give me something that helps me do my job better and faster, and I'll use it."

Specificity

An EHR 's capacity to adapt to the unique needs of different users is called specificity. A pediatrician, for example, serves different patients than a cardiologist (at least, we hope so) and naturally has different information requirements than a cardiologist. A good EHR is one that reconfigures itself to meet the specific needs of both physicians.

One popular way to build specificity into an EHR is to provide a "best of breed" system for each medical specialty. This approach has often been used in university hospitals, where each department is it's own fiefdom. The problem with this approach is that it can be very difficult and expensive to make the various specialty systems talk to one another. As a result, there have been a number of high-profile "best of breed" failures. The ideal EHR, by contrast, serves a pediatrician as well as it serves a cardiologist (or, for that matter, a family physician, general surgeon, or endocrinologist).

Fortunately, building in this degree of specificity isn't as difficult as it may sound. That's because there are really only two major differences between the specialties when it comes to an EHR. First, different clinical specialists are interested in slightly different parts of the chart. A cardiologist, for instance, may want to highlight EKG results while a pediatrician may be more interested in seeing a history of recent immunizations. Second, different specialists have different documentation requirements related to the services they provide.

The first issue—chart viewing—can be addressed by a system that offers customizable views of the clinical data stored in the database. The second issue—documentation—is addressed by built-in templates that guide physicians in entering a variety of different notes into the chart.

Workflow

Wander into the IT department of an organization that's implementing a new EHR system and chances are you'll hear at least one person say, "it's not about the software." That's the rallying cry of those who understand that the success or failure of an EHR hinges less on the software itself than on your ability to change, or re-engineer, common workflows that are inefficient. The EHR software is simply an enabler of more efficient work patterns; it can't make you work more efficiently. So the key to a successful implementation is your willingness to identify and fix outdated ways of accomplishing clinical work. If your organization isn't ready to clean house when it comes to workflows, then the EHR implementation will most likely fail. It's as simple as that.

Not surprisingly, then, the best EHRs are designed to be highly flexible around workflows. Again, this process is not as difficult as it might seem. Even though medicine is incredibly complex, the process of providing ambulatory care can be broken down into a finite number of workflows. Examples include medication renewal, taking care of a patient with an acute self-limited disease, managing diabetes, communicating test results back to a patient, and referring a patient to a different provider. As the organization identifies and re-designs its most common workflows, the EHR you choose should be configurable and able to support a variety of approaches to automating these tasks.

If that sounds obvious, consider that many EHR systems enable *incomplete* workflows, so that clinicians who use them to begin an automated task find they must switch to a manual process in the middle and then back again to the computer to finish up. Talk about frustrating! Needless to say, a good EHR is designed to accomplish common workflows from beginning to end on the computer.

Deployability

The healthcare industry is full of stories of EHRs that took more than five years to be fully implemented. That's at least five times longer than the organizations involved expected it would take. And yet, they could have shortened the deployment significantly if they had followed certain guidelines. For instance, one of the most common causes of a lengthy deployment is the mistaken belief that the best way to implement an EHR is to give a select group of tech-savvy physicians the entire suite of EHR functions ahead of everyone else. The thinking goes that once this group of early adopters has adjusted to using the EHR, a second group of physicians would then receive it, and so on until everyone was up and running on the system.

The problem with this scenario is that the early adopters are usually highly motivated and committed to making the system work, while later adopters are less motivated. Faced with the need to adjust to an entirely new way of practicing medicine overnight, these non-motivated physicians respond by refusing to use the complicated new system, thus delaying the entire implementation. Typically, after several years of this, only the early adopters and a handful of other physicians will still be using the EHR. This schism creates even more problems for the organization as it struggles to reconcile data from two vastly different systems—the old paper system and the new but rarely used EHR.

A much more rational approach is to incrementally deploy the EHR, starting by giving *all* physicians a small part of the new system and only adding more functions after they're comfortable using it. Giving physicians the easiest EHR functions first builds their confidence and lets them see that adopting the EHR is worth the effort. With that experience under their belts, most clinicians will be ready for and even excited about the next step.

VITALS

If you decide to deploy your EHR in increments, be sure to avoid vendors who offer an incremental approach but charge you for the entire system from day one. If you're doing an incremental deployment, then you should only have to pay for those portions of the system that are currently in use.

Scalability

The final item on our mental model's list of critical attributes is scalability. A highly scalable EHR serves both very large and very small clinics equally well. Why is scalability important? The needs of clinicians working in environments of different sizes are quite similar. The only reason clinicians in small practices may settle for a less robust system is price. Ideally, when an

EHR is designed correctly, it can serve practices of all sizes—the 600-physician integrated delivery network as well as the two-person family physician office.

You might wonder why this should be of interest to you. If you were in a large organization, would it be of use for you to be able to make your system available to smaller independent practices in your community? By offering to host the system for practices that couldn't otherwise afford a sophisticated system, you would be providing a real service. In return, you might find that hosting is a good way to expand your network of referral and referring physicians. Clinicians in a smaller setting may think that the only system they can afford will offer a mere shadow of the capability they want from an EHR. If a larger organization or perhaps an MSO or IPA were to offer to lease them access to a full EHR for a modest monthly fee, it might be the perfect solution. And, in fact, the hosted/ASP model for delivering EHR services is quickly becoming popular with health care organizations large and small.

Now let's turn to the main portion of the EHR Mental Model, the functionality you should consider when purchasing an EHR. As we discussed earlier, the inner square of the Mental Model diagram stands for an EHR's core capabilities, while the outer squares represent more advanced capabilities. It's important that you have a general understanding of both so that you can choose the right product and set reasonable expectations for your journey. This is true even if you intend to start with an incremental deployment that uses only the core functions.

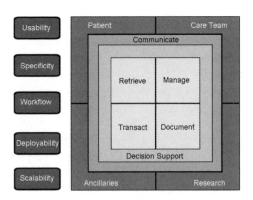

The EHR Mental Model

Core Functions of the EHR

At the very heart of the EHR are the functions *Retrieve, Transact, Manage,* and *Document.* If you're doing an incremental deployment, you might decide to begin by implementing only a subset of these four capabilities. But you won't be able to get rid of the paper chart until you incorporate all four.

When combined with *Decision-Support,* the four core components represent a reasonably complete electronic health record. So let's explore these components first and then turn our attention to the advanced functionality that we believe will drive universal adoption of the EHR in the United States.

Retrieve

The retrieve function allows users to find and view information that resides in the electronic record database. For many physicians, the primary motivation for adopting an EHR is the promise of having information about their patients instantly available at their fingertips. An excellent way to introduce busy clinicians to the value of the EHR is to implement only the retrieve function. It's an important first step that doesn't require major changes in behavior. In fact, physicians can continue to dictate or hand-write notes, prescriptions and orders which can then be scanned or typed into the EHR with the help of the clinical staff. Because it makes patients' charts ubiquitously accessible, the retrieve function is often enough to motivate clinicians to learn how to use the other core EHR functions.

Information retrieval does much more than simply put the patient's record onscreen. Physicians can greatly enhance the usefulness of the information they retrieve by applying any of three fundamental methods for viewing the information—automated patient summaries, trends and customized views. Each of these methods allows the user to choose how to view the contents of the electronic record, whether they're looking at office notes, lab tests, imaging results, consultations, nursing notes, visit slips, or insurance forms. The EHR lets users tailor their view of the patient's multi-faceted medical history to

> **VITALS**
>
> **An excellent way to introduce busy clinicians to the value of the EHR is to implement only the retrieve function. It's an important first step that delivers real value (instant access to patient information) without requiring major changes in behavior.**

provide either a comprehensive, all-in-one picture or to weed out unnecessary information and focus solely on the data they need to accomplish their particular goals.

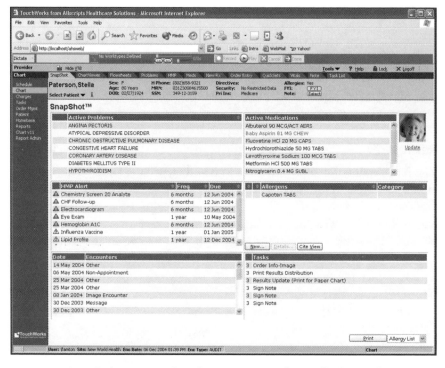

A typical automated patient summary of a medical record

Beyond the Face Sheet: The Automated Patient Summary

The automated patient summary is a snapshot of the record in a format that resembles (but improves upon) the first page of a paper chart, widely known as the "face sheet." It's a bit like having a table of contents for the full record. The automated patient summary in a typical EHR outlines the patient's current medical status, including medications, allergies, immunization status and a problem list. The value of the electronic summary is that it provides the entire organization with a concise, easy-to-read, high-level understanding of the patient's status. Since 80 percent of the value of a chart lies in only about 20 percent of its content, the automated patient summary's ability to encapsulate the most critical content is a truly high-value component of the EHR.

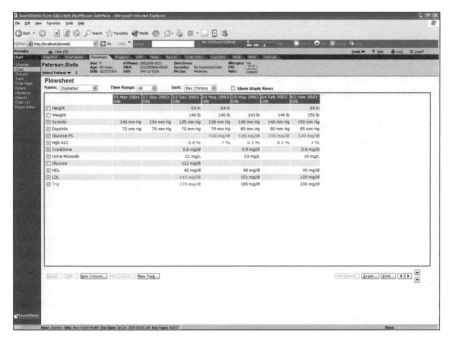

An EHR's Trend view of a typical patient's medical record

Trends

Data retrieved from the electronic record can also be viewed as a trend. Unlike the patient summary, which provides a static snapshot of the patient at one point in time, trends use flowcharts and graphs to track the patient's progress over time. This capability is especially useful for tracking the progress of patients with chronic problems such as diabetes. Unfortunately, creating the charts by hand is time consuming and difficult. Someone has to physically maintain the flowchart as well as document a note for each visit. Not so with the EHR, which can create and update flowcharts in a matter of microseconds.

VITALS

The EHR can be configured to automatically maintain predefined flowcharts that are instantly updated whenever a new test result, vital sign or note is entered into the system. EHR flowcharts can be the tool of choice for quickly tracking a particular set of objective findings, symptoms or tests across a series of patient visits.

Practice-Specific Filtering

The third way that the EHR supports retrieving information from the electronic record is by allowing each user to electronically filter the contents of the chart to meet their particular needs. For instance, a cardiologist working in a large multi-specialty group might want to gather in one place, electronically, a summary of all the documents and test results generated within that specialty. A family physician, on the other hand, might want to organize the chart contents by medical problem, while an internist might set up the EHR to mimic the sections and subsections in the paper record. In each case, the EHR is able to organize the details of the chart and its individual "pages" in a highly specific, customized manner. It's something you just couldn't do with the paper record.

In addition to tailoring the contents of the record to their specific needs, clinicians can easily use the EHR to search for particular results or notes. For example, the clinician could quickly look up all hospital discharge summaries for the past year to assess patterns of serious exacerbations in her patients' chronic illnesses.

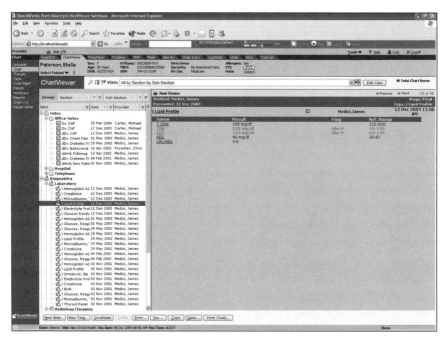

EHRs let clinicians customize how they view the medical record

Each of these capabilities is a clear improvement over the paper record, which not only doesn't provide customized views but requires users to page through information they don't need to get to the information they do. More, the EHR's enhanced record-retrieval and viewing capabilities are available to everyone in the organization, no matter where they are. Support staff no longer has to track down the paper record or, worse, depend on a duplicative and perhaps inaccurate "ghost copy" of the record.

Transact

The second core function of an EHR refers to the clinical process of creating electronic orders, prescriptions, referrals, customized patient-education materials and other administrative tools that support therapeutic medicine. With a paper record, these transactions typically begin with users filling out forms and end in a manual communication of some kind (e.g., sending a prescription to the pharmacy or an order to the lab). No matter which way you look at it, *transact* is a critical part of medical care. In the pre-electronic paper world, it's where most medical errors begin and so is the biggest source of potential harm to patients. It is also the starting point of most medical costs. Nearly 80 cents out of every dollar spent in healthcare originates with a transaction that declares a clinician's decision—whether it is a prescription for a chronic medication, a series of lab tests or an order for a diagnostic image.

Transact also is the point at which decision-support is most critical (and electronic decision support the most successful). There is no better time for clinicians to refer to best practices than when they are preparing to write orders or prescriptions, or proposing a diagnostic or therapeutic procedure.

> **VITALS**
>
> **The benefits of electronic orders and prescriptions vs. paper:**
>
> - less prone to error
> - faster
> - more reliable
> - more easily tracked for quality assurance
> - includes information about cost and insurance coverage.

And yet, even physicians who use an EHR for other purposes often avoid using one to generate clinical transactions. Most prefer to give verbal orders to a nurse who then handles the transaction. The problem with the verbal approach is that the clinician misses the opportunity to be informed about the best decision via electronic decision-support tools.

Manage

The management of patients over time is the third core function of an EMR, one that is especially well suited to the ambulatory setting. Ambulatory care differs from acute care not only in treating less severe conditions but also in monitoring patients over a period of weeks or years rather than days. This long-term treatment is often coordinated across a team of caregivers including the primary care physician and any required specialists. In addition to management of acute, self-limited problems, ambulatory care focuses on health maintenance—doing what is necessary to prevent illness—and chronic disease management—doing what is appropriate and cost-effective to minimize the impact of chronic illness on the patient's quality of life.

The EHR can be a tremendous aid for ambulatory clinicians who manage patients over time. An HMP (Health Management Plan) tool, for instance, can assign and track periodic events such as routine mammograms or a glycohemoglobin test for diabetics. The HMP helps assure that critical tests and procedures don't fall through the cracks. It also can assist the administrative staff in notifying patients about upcoming appointments.

Tools to assist in referrals are another example of the management function of an EMR. Consultants who work in the same organization as the primary care doctor can receive electronic consultation requests linked to the patient's electronic record. That speeds an understanding of the patient and minimizes expensive duplicate tests. Once the consultation report is ready, it can automatically be emailed to the primary care doctor and any other clinicians who need to see it.

Other important examples of the management function are the electronic medication and problem lists. Problems can be annotated, modified and shared among the team of physicians caring for a patient. And the medication list serves as the basis for automatic medication renewals and for tracking the benefit or lack of benefit from various medications (information that can also be useful for a system-wide cost-benefit analysis).

Document

The fourth and final core function is what most clinicians think of when they hear the terms EHR or EMR. The *document* function lets physicians capture their thoughts and actions during a patient encounter and assemble them into a formal clinical document or office note.

Documenting the encounter is one of the most onerous tasks in clinical practice. For the past 100 years doctors have been obligated to keep what is essentially a diary of everything they do with each and every patient. Even more frustrating, much of the documenting that clinicians do is redundant because the same information appears in different parts of the paper chart. Nonetheless, their notes must be laboriously handwritten or dictated—the latter at significant expense.

Thankfully, the EHR promises to greatly simplify clinical documentation and reduce the cost of transcription. The catch is that previous documentation systems have generally been so complicated that they're difficult for users to learn and difficult to operate with speed. Given the choice between a new, complicated process that takes twice as long as their current method, clinicians will opt for the habitual one every time.

It doesn't have to be that way. Clinical documentation on a computer can be just as fast or faster than manual methods, depending on the quality of the system. The mark of a robust EHR is its ability to adapt to a number of different documentation approaches. For instance, the system should be able to automatically document what it already "knows" about the patient. Once the clinician has dictated the medication or problem list, it should never have to be dictated again. Recent results should be automatically cited in the note, when desired, as should any orders, prescriptions, or additions to the problem list. And clinicians who currently dictate should be able to dictate portions of a note and have the EHR automatically insert the information where it belongs. (This is an effective way to reduce the cost of transcription without forcing clinicians to change all of their habits). Finally, a robust EHR should let the clinician type the note or else use handwriting recognition with text macros on a tablet computer to enter short, common phrases.

Another beneficial capability of a good EHR is structured charting. Using this approach, clinicians build a description of the patient's history or physical status from a series of standardized menus or "pick lists" of clinical terms. Ideally, the pick list contains standard discrete terms such as those found in SNOMED or MEDCIN. Because it is standardized, the resulting note is searchable, offering significantly more functionality. Notably, the system can use the pick list terms to calculate an Evaluation and Management (E&M) code for the patient visit—a task that becomes far more difficult when using a dictation or text macro.

Structured charting is controversial, however, for the same reason that digital documentation is—the process can be difficult to learn and slow to operate. Moreover, given the dizzying array of symptoms or physical findings that patients can present with, it takes a lot of work to set up a computer to sequentially display the proper pick lists (a series of standardized menus of clinical terms that define the contents of the chart). Still, with a little effort, many physicians find that structured charting can be almost as fast as paper charting and far more functional.

In the near future, we expect that EHRs will come equipped with affordable and accurate Natural Language Processing that can extract meaning from dictated or typed text. That would give clinicians the best of both worlds—a searchable, automatically coded clinical record that could be created using a combination of voice recognition and typed or dictated notes.

VITALS

Voice recognition, the Holy Grail of documentation, is here at last. After years of disappointing performance, voice recognition software today is good enough to benefit large numbers of physicians. A robust EHR can incorporate voice recognition seamlessly into the clinical note.

The Middle Ground: Decision Support

Let's return to the diagram of the EHR Mental Model for a look at *decision support*, the system's ability to help clinicians make better judgments. A decade ago, that capability was idealistically dubbed "artificial intelligence" and many worried that computers would soon co-opt the physician's decision-making role. After it became apparent that true AI was at best a distant dream, the industry coined the term "decision support" to reflect more realistic expectations.

Decision support has a number of different operations, the most common of which is the simple alert. Alerts are automatic pop-up messages that warn of potentially adverse consequences if the clinician continues with an action such as prescribing a drug that is known to be dangerous in combination with another drug the patient is taking. Supporters of alerts laud their ability to prevent not only harmful decisions but inappropriately costly ones as well. For instance, alerts can prevent clinicians from ordering diagnostic tests that have already been ordered by another clinician. But critics of alerts warn that it can be difficult for clinicians to determine whether they are appropriate or not. Many drug interactions, for example, are already well known to physicians. Drug-related alerts that pop up too frequently tend to discourage busy physicians from paying attention to alerts.

Another type of decision-support is called "referential decision-support." This method focuses on ensuring that the information needed to make good decisions is always close at hand. For example, a clinician can voluntarily call up a short monograph describing the appropriate use of a medication before prescribing it. Or he can access evidence-based guidelines that come in useful chunks of information appropriate to the clinical context. The advantage of referential decision-support is that it puts the physician in the driver's seat. Because he must make a conscious choice to seek the additional information rather than having it forced upon him by an alert, he may be more likely to pay attention to it. We expect decision-support to become more sophisticated and effective as EHRs become more widely utilized.

> **VITALS**
>
> In its landmark reports on medical safety, "To Err is Human," and "Crossing the Quality Chasm," The Institute of Medicine notes that while we lack evidence about the best way to treat every illness, the essence of safety is consistently following guidelines that we *know* work. The EHR makes it easier for clinicians to do just that.

Extending the EHR Beyond the Office

Returning again to the diagram of the EHR Mental Model, you'll notice that the outer quadrants (Patient, Care Team, Research and Ancillaries) are nearly a mirror image of the inner quadrants (Retrieve, Manage, Document, Transact). Their common boundary is the interface between Decision-Support and Communicate. While the inner squares represent the core of the EHR—functions used by the clinician during a patient encounter—the outer portion represents the extension of the EHR beyond the physician-patient in-office dyad. The core EHR has the potential to vastly improve clinical efficiency, consistency and quality. The outer quadrants have the potential to transform healthcare as we know it. They embody the future—in fact, a relatively *near* future, if large group practices continue to adopt the EHR at their current pace.

Let's run through the elements of the Mental Model's outer quadrant one by one.

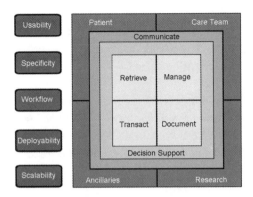

The EHR Mental Model

The Patient

You can't blame patients for assuming that healthcare revolves around them. That's certainly how it would work in an ideal universe. The truth, however, is far more prosaic: Today's healthcare system was designed principally to serve the physician. Patients must adapt to their doctor's schedule, cede control over their personal health information, and expect to receive only that information which their doctor chooses to reveal to them.

At least, that was the case before the arrival of the Internet. The information age, coupled with dramatic shifts in the way services are reimbursed, is producing patients who behave more like traditional free-market consumers than the passive consenters the system was designed to manage. Like all consumers, today's healthcare consumers demand good value, which generally means quick, easy access to the latest in medical science, and doctors who keep them fully informed about their health options.

The EHR can rapidly accelerate the process of using technology to turn health consumers into fully empowered partners on the healthcare team. One of the most powerful forces in changing patient behavior is the advice they receive from a respected physician. Linking physicians and patients together via the EHR and its associated eHealth applications has huge potential for enhancing the trust and respect inherent in their relationship.

A good example of the EHR's eHealth functionality is the Portable Health Record (also known as a Personal Health Record), which lets patients access a subset of the information their care team sees. In most cases, patients using a PHR can retrieve an accurate list of their active medications, allergies, problems, important lab test results and maybe even the progress notes created by their providers. The "portability" part of PHR refers to the patient's ability to make their digital clinical information available to the physicians of their choice.

Other popular EHR eHealth functions include eMessaging and eVisits. Both enable patients, physicians and other members of the care team to communicate about particular health issues via secure electronic messaging. Popular uses include automated requests for medication-renewal, post-visit follow-up questions, or engaging the physician in an electronic dialog in place of an office visit. Some insurance companies are currently experimenting with paying for eVisits and a growing number of physicians offer both services to patients on a self-paid basis.

Another intriguing eHealth feature is the ability to interview patients online and use the information to gauge the appropriateness of appointment requests as well as to speed documentation. Such a process begins when a patient develops, say, a persistent cough and phones (or eMessages) to request an office visit. Using the EHR, the office staff could immediately send the patient an automated questionnaire that would ask most of the questions a clinician would ask about the cough. The results would be sent to a nurse for confirmation that the visit is appropriate. They could also be automatically incorporated into the physician's note, thus significantly reducing clinician time spent on the subjective portion of the note. Even more intriguing is the notion of using such patient interviewing software to close the loop on outcomes. Based on the patients' care plan, the EHR could automatically email them questions designed to discover if their health improved or worsened following therapy.

Each of these eHealth initiatives can be performed using today's technology. What's been missing is the imperative within healthcare organizations to make it happen. That imperative is fast developing as more and more HCOs experience the improvements that come from eHealth. In fact, we predict that eHealth will soon be as widespread as eCommerce, and that the 21st century in healthcare will be known as the "Age of the Patient." eHealth is so clearly the wave of the future that we believe it is a critical component to look for when shopping for an EHR.

The Care Team

Just as the EHR can enhance the care team's communications with patients and vice versa, it also can improve the team's internal coordination. From the patient's perspective, better coordination among all the health professionals involved in her care would be ideal. No one would then have to ask her twice for the same information, or order tests that had already been done. And the entire care team would immediately be advised when new information suggested a change in her therapy.

Unfortunately, team coordination is clearly not optimal in today's healthcare system. Ask yourself how many times you've seen a patient treated in the emergency department and then referred back to their primary care physician without a record of what transpired there. Wouldn't it be great if ambulatory care clinicians could electronically incorporate key summary documents from the hospital into the ambulatory record? Wouldn't care be enhanced if hospital-based physicians could electronically access a summary of the ambulatory record to aid them in creating an admitting history and physical?

The number of everyday situations that could benefit from better care-team coordination is nearly unlimited. The solution lies in finding the root cause of the coordination problem. Healthcare workers are strongly motivated to improve coordination, so the problem doesn't lie with them. The real culprit is the old paper-based management systems that make distributed care teams far more difficult to manage. Fortunately, information technology is beginning to change that. A top-notch EHR has at its heart an intra-office communication engine that operates much like an intelligent email program. The intra-office engine can link email messages from any care-team member, whether ambulatory or hospital-based, with the appropriate components of the chart and so coordinate tasks such as renewal of medications, review of consultation notes and appropriate responses to patient phone calls.

Thanks to a pair of federal initiatives known as the National Health Information Infrastructure (NHII) and the Regional Health Information Organizations, EHR care-team coordination should expand beyond the individual office or health system within the next decade. The federal technology initiatives, which will be overseen by the US Office of the National Coordinator for Health Information Technology, promise to connect every part of the national healthcare system. Clinicians would then have access to every patient's full medical record, regardless of where that information was collected. By bringing patient records and prescriptions out of the realm of ink and paper, the new HIT initiatives are expected to facilitate improvements not only in healthcare coordination but also in overall safety, quality and efficiency.

Ancillaries

The next outer quadrant in the EHR Mental Model concerns communication with systems peripheral to the core healthcare team. Such ancillary systems include laboratories as well as a rapidly growing army of health technology devices that can be used directly by patients. A graphic example of these new devices is the popular Japanese "smart toilet," now available in the US, which can perform automated urinalysis, pulse and blood pressure checks. Sporting modems, the smart toilets can act as an early warning system of emerging health problems. A homegrown and slightly larger example of the same trend is the new "smart home" being developed at the Massachusetts Institute of Technology and elsewhere. The wired and wireless homes fulfill one of the ultimate promises of health IT—its ability to better manage chronic disease by enabling patients to interact with home-based monitors and therapeutic devices. The EHR of the near future will communicate with all of these devices through standardized interfaces. When combined with patient-interviewing software and other eHealth components, these emerging tools will revolutionize the way we treat the most common and costly chronic diseases.

Research

The final quadrant in the EHR Mental Model, healthcare research, will also benefit from the widespread adoption of the EHR, broad use of eHealth and a national healthcare IT infrastructure. Here are just a few examples to get your imagination going:

Enhanced drug trials. Physicians' groups with an EHR can substantially boost revenue by providing services to pharmaceutical companies. The drug firms pay a premium for EHR-enabled services like finding good candidates for drug trials and managing patients who are taking emerging medications. And with genomics on the horizon, the expected explosion in drug research will require even more refined case finding—something the EHR is ideally suited for.

> **VITALS**
>
> When combined with the National Health Information Infrastructure, the EHR will be able to automatically aggregate adverse drug reactions across the nation. For the first time, pharmaceutical companies and the FDA will have real-time data on the efficacy of new drugs.

Real-time, proactive outcomes research. As we discussed earlier, eHealth holds the promise of instantly tracking the efficacy of any therapy, even for the most routine problems. Now for the first time healthcare systems can gather the long-coveted outcomes data on routine care. By aggregating the data regionally and even nationally, the EHR will expand the body of medical knowledge and provide new evidence for determining appropriate care.

Meaningful quality comparisons. Increasingly market-driven, the healthcare system is rapidly embracing a pay-for-performance model that requires organizations to prove their care exceeds emerging quality standards. In this new world, the EHR can play a dual role. On the one hand, it enables HCOs to easily track, analyze and demonstrate their outcomes data. On the other hand, the EHR in combination with the NHII will provide an even more potent tool for plans, employers and government to objectively compare HCOs' performance. Some find this prospect scary; others find it empowering. But whether you like it or not, the future of health care will be one of increasing transparency and meaningful competition based on quality and outcomes. We can only hope that future payment schemes will reward providers based on quality rather than the arbitrary regional model now practiced by Medicare and others.

The Recap

- The most critical element of any EHR is its usability. To appeal to its intended users, an EHR must first provide a positive user experience, which in turn requires an intuitive learning process, easy-to-retain directions, and flexibility in accommodating a variety of pathways to performing tasks.

- The success or failure of an EHR hinges less on the software itself than on your ability to change, or re-engineer, common workflows that are inefficient. The EHR software is simply an enabler of more efficient work patterns; it can't make you work more efficiently. So the key to a successful implementation is your willingness to identify and fix outdated ways of accomplishing clinical work.

- At the very heart of the EHR are the functions *Retrieve, Transact, Manage,* and *Document.* If you're doing an incremental deployment, you might decide to begin by implementing only a subset of these four capabilities. But you won't be able to get rid of the paper chart until you incorporate all four.

- While we lack evidence about the best way to treat every illness, the essence of safety is consistently following guidelines that we *know* work. The EHR makes it easier for clinicians to do just that by providing electronic decision support capabilities.

- The core EHR—those functions used by the clinician during a patient encounter—has the potential to vastly improve clinical efficiency, consistency and quality. Yet the EHR is also capable of extending care beyond the physician-patient in-office dyad. If healthcare organizations continue to adopt the EHR at their current rate, it can be expected to radically transform healthcare as we know it.

If You Have Time

- The Computer-Based Patient Record: An Essential Technology for Healthcare. Richard Dick, Elaine B. Steen and Don Detmer. National Academy Press; 1st edition (January 15, 1997).

- Information Systems for Healthcare Management, Sixth Edition. Charles J. Austin, Stuart B. Boxerman. Health Administration Press; 6th edition (December 1, 2002).

- The CEO's Guide to Health Care Information Systems, 2nd Edition. Joseph M. DeLuca, Rebecca Enmark. Jossey-Bass; 2nd edition (September 14, 2001).

CHAPTER THREE

Driving Physician Adoption Through Physician-Centric Design

In This Chapter
- Find and train physician leaders
- Understand the stages of technology adoption
- Build and load appropriate content
- Drive physician adoption

Perhaps the most important piece in the EHR implementation puzzle is knowing how to create and configure a system that systematically addresses the needs of physicians. This chapter will outline a plan for accomplishing that goal by getting physicians deeply involved in and committed to the implementation. It will explore the normal stages of technology adoption in an effort to understand how and why physicians react to the EHR. This understanding, in turn, will inform your implementation strategy, as well as determine how you will work with physicians to gain their acceptance and, ultimately, their adoption of this technology. Finally, the chapter will examine content loading from the physician's perspective.

Developing Physician Leaders: How to Empower Physicians to be Effective Change Agents

An EHR implementation is not just another IT project. As the EHR's clinical tools become more sophisticated and more organizations use them to eliminate the paper record, implementations increasingly require substantial and meaningful participation by clinicians. While they may initially resist the implementation—change is scary, after all—once physician leaders recognize that implementing an EHR is imminent, they'll want a significant voice in the process.

In fact, physicians increasingly are becoming active change agents who drive the decision to acquire an EHR. This has long been the case for the few small independent practices that spend their own money to purchase a system. However, most large organizations that installed an EHR in the past had to drag clinicians into the process kicking, screaming and clutching their paper charts and Dictaphones. That is rarely the case today. Once projects get under way, clinicians in even the largest organizations tend to request a role in determining how the system is implemented.

While physicians are becoming more interested in EHR implementations, their busy schedules mean they generally get involved late in the project. By then, the project team has fought hard to gain control over the implementation and physician demands may spark a crippling power struggle. Your challenge is to find a way to identify, train and involve key physicians earlier in the process and to nurture a constructive working relationship between them and your project team. Without such a relationship, the implementation may be doomed.

Why? Today's second- and third-generation EHR systems offer sophisticated clinical capabilities that require considerable clinical input, process design and ongoing support. Ideally, physicians will drive the content and clinical workflow enhancements that are at the heart of an EHR implementation. Favorites lists, note templates, and order item dictionaries are just a few of the content-building tasks that demand substantial clinical involvement and commitment. The project team's role should be to teach, assist, encourage and provide operational and IT support to the physician leaders in this effort.

As outlined in Chapter Seven (Building and Managing Effective Project Teams), the project's executive leadership should ideally consist of an Executive Sponsor and a primary Physician Sponsor who together help define the expected

VITALS

Doctors respond best to persuasive arguments that mirror their own clinical evaluation processes. When attempting to champion the EHR, use authoritative arguments that appeal to empirical evidence, such as peer-reviewed studies proving its clinical benefits. Back up your arguments with site visits to demonstrate your interest.

outcomes and ensure that organizational support is strong for the other components of the project team structure. The primary Physician Sponsor, therefore, plays a lead role in the project even before the creation of the project team.

Besides the primary Physician Sponsor, each clinic or location where the EHR will be implemented should have one or more local Physician Champions—influential physicians who are energized learners eager to share their knowledge with the clinic's end users. These local champions will assist in the management of change at each location or clinic through their involvement in the review of the system design and validation of the system configuration. The Project Manager will rely on their local knowledge to determine the project's timing, to uncover potential risks and identify key influencers in their clinics. As Chapter Seven describes, soliciting the participation of this small group of Physician Champions is a powerful mechanism to affect change at the clinic level.

(Because the following guidelines apply to the primary Physician Sponsor as well as Physician Champions, to avoid confusion we will dispense with the formal team titles and refer to both roles as "physician leaders").

Identifying Potential Leaders

How do you identify and grow physician leaders within your organization? The first step is to be clear what you mean by a physician leader. Ironically, the right leader for an EHR implementation is rarely a computer enthusiast, because other physicians are likely to dismiss this physician's enthusiasm for the EHR as enthusiasm for computerized solutions in general. Ideally, physician leaders are solution agnostic—that is, they are interested in improving clinical quality and efficiency, and willing to investigate any tool that may help. Physician leaders also need to be respected peers—good clinicians with an interest in process improvement. They need to be good communicators and, ideally, good teachers. As a rule of thumb, you can look for leaders among those who show an interest in exploring new ways of doing business.

Unfortunately, potential physician leaders are often so weighed down by the daily work of clinical practice that they haven't had the opportunity to shine. A large, transformative project like an EHR implementation is the perfect opportunity to develop clinician leaders. In searching for the best candidates, recognize that not everyone who expresses interest will work out. It can be particularly difficult to resist the enthusiasm and energy of physician computer geeks vying for a role. While you may be forced to include a geek on your team, make an effort to find and encourage less fervent physicians who have demonstrated leadership on other projects.

Aim to have at least one physician leader for every 25-30 physicians in your organization. The goal of your sponsors is to actively participate in the design and development phases of the project, to become the initial "super users" of the system, to support and encourage their fellow physicians, and ultimately to help develop additional super users. A super user is someone who not only knows the system backwards and forward but also is able to creatively adapt the system to his or her particular workflow goals. The Physician Sponsor and all Physician Champions are expected to be super-users, but others may earn the title as well. These can include nurses, supervisors, office managers, and anyone else in a role of some authority within the clinics or other locations where the new system will be implemented.

A common mistake is to expect physician leaders to carry a full clinical workload while they play a key role in driving the implementation's success. Yet physician leaders are so critical to a successful EHR implementation that it makes sense for the organization to lighten their clinical load. How much time each sponsor will need to fully devote to the project is a function of the number of sponsors and your particular implementation strategy. Rapid, "big bang" implementations require a huge time commitment on the part of sponsors, while a more incremental and phased rollout requires considerably less time. Either way, there is real work to be done, and it is very difficult to find time to do that work while carrying a full clinical load. We have found that the cost of freeing up some of your physician leaders' time is offset by their contribution to more rapid and effective physician utilization of the EHR, which is a key factor in generating a return on investment from the system.

Training Physician Leaders

How can you develop physician super users and champions reliably and cost-effectively? If it were practical, you would simply send them off to a three-week intensive training. But since hefty time commitments are probably out of the question, a fair compromise is to conduct two all-day training sessions for your initial group of sponsors. It's critical that these initial trainings be conducted offsite (and ideally led by the EHR vendor) because clinicians cannot concentrate while they are physically near the clinical environment; the temptation to combine training with ongoing clinical care is simply too great.

The first training can be done in conjunction with the training of the project team. Project team training happens very early in the implementation process and sometimes months before any users go live (for more details on project team training, see Chapter Ten). The training is intended to help the team learn enough about the EHR to be able to knowledgeably guide the implementation. Clinicians need a solid understanding of the system's capabilities before they can begin building the configuration and content for the organization. Your clinicians and project team will learn the basics of the system together, and this experience of going through boot camp together can build a lasting mutual respect that will benefit the overall project. This is also the time to set expectations about the roles that each group will play in the implementation.

(Note that not every topic in this first training program will be interesting to both groups; some of the initial project team training will be technical in nature and of little interest to the clinicians. Clinicians can use the time to hold breakout sessions that focus on the unique issues of teaching, encouraging and supporting their fellow physicians).

If your organization works with physicians from several different groups, this initial training will allow the clinicians to intermingle and produce a powerful cross-pollination of ideas. Most EHR trainers say they learn as much from these interactions as the students. You should encourage your physician leaders to form relationships with clinicians from other practices. Often the informal support networks they form can be an invaluable ongoing resource long after the class is finished.

The second offsite training for physician leaders should occur at the optimal "teachable moment." Such moments tend to occur after the student has taken their classroom training and put it to work in the field. That's because the best students are those who are motivated by an immediate and practical need for the subject being taught. For this reason, it's best to bring the sponsors back for advanced training after they have used major portions of the system in the field for at least one month. This will be a class devoted entirely to physician leaders. The curriculum includes a combination of product tricks and shortcuts, in-depth training on the art of creating templates for notes, as well as additional discussion on physician leadership and strategies for achieving clinician buy-in. Although EHR products may vary, this approach is universally applicable.

Of key importance is the teaching of EHR "art and strategy." For example, it's relatively easy to learn how to create a simple spreadsheet. However, figuring out how to solve a complex business problem using a spreadsheet requires knowledge of a different order. One of the best ways to acquire this knowledge is to study how other people have solved similar problems. The advanced training workshop should focus on the pros and cons of a variety of solutions to different clinical problems. For instance, one might approach the design of note templates differently for pediatric well child visits versus a multi-problem internal medicine visit. The template doesn't just contain different information and sections—it needs to be designed in a way that reflects the working habits of these two very different specialties.

Once the training of the physician leaders is complete, we suggest you (or your vendor) consider issuing a certificate stating that the clinician has achieved a particular level of mastery. These officially acknowledged clinicians are a valuable asset for the organization and vendor both. For example, certified leaders can be invaluable in providing feedback regarding system design, ideas for new features, and support for reviewing and editing new content in the product.

Stages of Technology Adoption

The introduction of any new technology brings new challenges along with new opportunities. Remember how awkward you felt using an ATM machine for the first time? That awkward response to the unfamiliar is part of the challenge. More recently, supermarkets have begun installing automatic checkout machines. Do you find yourself avoiding this new technology in favor of the more familiar checkout person? It turns out that the adoption of new technologies follows a predictable pattern that progresses from early resistance to radical transformation. It's helpful to understand this pattern because it can help explain users' responses to the EHR and therefore inform a rational approach to implementation.

Classical change-management theory identifies three phases that we all go through following the introduction of a new technology—the Substitutive, Innovative and Transformative phases of adoption.

The Substitutive Phase

The typical first reaction to a new technology is to substitute it in your mind for the technology it replaces. For instance, when the automobile was introduced in the early 20th century, the major mode of transportation was the horse and carriage. Not surprisingly, the first automobiles were called "horseless carriages." Clearly, people of the time could only picture the new technology through the lens of the old technology.

The substitutive phase fulfills an important role by helping people transition from the familiar to the new. It keeps us in our comfort zone when we are confronted by change. However, this phase of technology adoption is also limiting because it's difficult for people to achieve the full promise of a new technology when they are hobbled by the limitations of the old. For example, many people felt that the first automobiles were inferior to the horse and carriage, and they weren't far wrong. The infrastructure of the day was designed to supply hay, oats and water, not gasoline, and the roads were so poor that early cars often got stuck in conditions carriages managed just fine. These failings of comparison led many to avoid adopting the automobile, even though it offered several practical advantages over the horse and carriage.

There is an important lesson here for the EHR. The term electronic medical record is in itself substitutive for a paper medical record. Physicians who are stuck in the substitutive response to the new computerized record are unable to visualize the profound improvements to quality and efficiency that it promises to deliver. They are blinded by their allegiance to the safe and familiar paper record. A number of vendors have capitalized on this shortsighted response by designing systems that purposely resemble the paper record. These systems have the advantage of feeling familiar but because they fail to guide clinicians into the next two phases of technology adoption, their use leads to a safe but extremely limited functionality.

To avoid the substitutive trap, your organization's implementation strategy should help clinicians experience and then move as quickly as possible through this phase. If your system supports an incremental implementation (that is, one module at a time), you might consider implementing a first phase that includes the entire electronic chart (e.g., labs, dictated notes, scanned documents, etc.), but doesn't require clinicians to enter the information directly in the computer. This "electronic chart" is easy for most physicians to understand, because it is similar to but more convenient than the paper process they're accustomed to. It's substitutive in nature and relatively non-threatening, but it is different enough to encourage many of your physicians to say, "this is great—when can we do more?" Keep your ears open for that question. When you hear it, your clinicians are entering the second phase of technology adoption—the innovative.

The Innovative Phase

The innovative phase begins the moment your users start to become creative with the system. Once they become comfortable with the notion of an electronic chart, it becomes more obvious how the technology could help improve their lives. We should note that many of your leaders will understand this intuitively even before you begin the project. However, theoretical understanding and knowledge based on real experience are not the same. It is necessary to begin actual usage of the system and to go through a period of awkwardness (which can be short) before your old habits begin to be rewired, allowing for improvisation.

> **VITALS**
>
> Physicians, like other professionals, use an autonomous process to assess the value of new innovations. They first consider it, then test it, if possible, for its utility and cost, and finally make a deliberate decision to adopt or discard the approach.

During the innovative phase, your organization will begin to reap significant benefits from the EHR. Clinician users will naturally begin to tinker with ever-faster ways to document complex visits, make improvements to medication management, and build in automated quality initiatives. Your clinicians now begin to recognize how taking the time to become proficient in electronic prescribing can dramatically simplify the onerous medication renewal process.

Another hallmark of the innovative stage is the development of "systems thinking." Normally, clinicians are focused solely on getting their own work done as efficiently as possible, regardless of how their processes may impact the organization. When they adopt systems thinking, they consider the impact of their workflows on the efficiency of the entire organization. Because the innovative phase encourages systems thinking and organizational innovation, it can lead to dramatic improvements in efficiency and quality. Once an organization achieves critical mass in this phase, nothing can stop their success. The advanced clinician training mentioned earlier is one of the key steps in generating this critical mass.

The Transformative Phase

You'll recognize that you have reached the final, transformative phase of technology adoption when you realize you're doing things with the new technology that you couldn't have imagined doing when you started your journey. Transformation is the magic that happens when we evolve to our next level of understanding. It can't happen without a period of innovation, trial and error. But given time, transformation is inevitable. Think of how your life has been changed by the Internet. Few of those who used the first, crude e-mail programs in the early '90s imagined they would one day routinely use e-mail as part of their jobs. Talk to anyone who has been using an EHR for two or three years and you'll find that they've experienced a similar transformation and have accomplished far more than they set out to accomplish.

On the macro level, the transformative phase is the critical step that every healthcare organization must take if it is to remain competitive and viable in today's marketplace. It's unlikely that the problems with the American healthcare system are going to be fixed by business as usual, or incremental improvements. Most observers agree that we need to find a way to re-invent healthcare in America, which is another way of expressing the notion of transformation. Transforming or re-inventing the way you do business is a worthy justification for introducing information technology into your organization. The good news is that if you work through the substitutive phase and consciously encourage innovation, you will indeed wake up one day to realize that you have transformed your organization.

Content Loading: Strategies for Making the System Make Sense to Physicians

In addition to teaching other physicians about the EHR and designing more efficient workflows, physician leaders play a critical role in assuring that the system makes sense to clinicians from the first day they use it. Just as the substitutive phase of your project should be designed to ease the transition from old habits to a new way of doing business, one of the project team's most important jobs is to maximize physician comfort with the new system by ensuring that the content is familiar and complete. Content loading may be the single most important factor in achieving physician buy-in and utilization during the substitutive phase. (For more discussion of content loading, see Chapter Eight, which discusses processes for converting existing digital information into EHR content).

Two of the most important types of content are pick lists and patient content. Pick lists are the options the system gives a user for completing a task, presented as a series of standardized menus of clinical terms. For example, effective e-prescribing products generally provide the clinician with a list of the most common ways they have written prescriptions in the past. This makes it much easier for the clinician to rapidly write prescriptions on the computer. Without these condensed lists, the clinician would have to find the drug from a list of thousands, and then specify a customized sig—a chore that would surely convince physicians stuck in the substitutive phase that "the old way was better."

Patient content refers to the nuts and bolts of the electronic record—every piece of information that completes the electronic record, from lists of medications, problems and allergies to lab data and notes. The project team must ensure that clinicians are introduced to an EHR already populated with enough patient data to be of real value. For example, when a clinician first uses the system, if he has to manually enter a medication list for each patient, he will soon become discouraged because of the extra time required. By developing strategies for populating the record with current, complete data, the project team ensures that clinicians are introduced to a robust and truly useful system.

Your physician leaders will need to roll up their sleeves and coordinate consensus for pick lists and note templates among their peers. It is important that doctors in your organization have the opportunity to provide input into these lists. Once consensus is reached, the work of creating pick lists and patient content can be partially automated. For example, some vendors make it possible to pull all medications known to insurance companies (via PBMs) into the electronic chart. This provides a huge head start in building patient medication lists. Lists of common diagnoses for each specialty can be obtained from specialty organizations as well as claims data from your practice management system.

Unfortunately, the process can't always be automated. For that reason, organizations should seriously consider assigning staff to enter problems and allergies from the paper chart. To avoid overload, start with those patients who have appointments in the next day or two.

Some EHR vendors create a Clinical Content Library (CCL) that lets customers share the content they have created. Your vendor should offer this service or at least provide a starter kit of content as well as a strategy for creating appropriate initial patient content. Ideally the content library should make it easy to import the best-practices data for any particular specialty, provide a way for customers to share their experience, and allow them to rate the available content.

Many organizations leave content development to the project team, but larger organizations should consider hiring a clinical person to support the physician leaders in managing this activity. One organization addressed this issue by assigning responsibility for content development to a full-time nurse who works as part of the physician leaders team to solicit feedback from other physicians. The nurse builds and manages updates to the system's content, acting in the capacity of EHR librarian—definitely not a job for a non-clinical person.

Finally, as a guiding principle in nurturing your physician leaders, managing the stages of technology adoption, and building appropriate content, always keep in mind the principle of IDDUINEM—If Doctors Don't Use It, Nothing Else Matters. This principal, which is true in all cases, suggests you should devote a substantial portion of the creative energy spent on the project to developing strategies for gaining early and persistent physician involvement and commitment to success. This chapter has focused on several of those strategies but they are merely a starting point for your own creative process. If you have a clear goal—such as universal and effective clinician utilization—you will surely find many other creative ways to make it happen.

VITALS

Clinical content loading tips:

- Populate the charts with the problem and medication lists before scanning documents into the EHR (it's mechanically easier than doing it after scanning).
- Load clinical data prior to the patient's appointment. For instance, load the next day's problem and medication lists or the next week's patient information from the appointment schedule.
- Hire temporary nurses to perform content loading or use MAs.
- Increase appointment times by 10 minutes for a couple of months to allow nurses to enter the data during triage.

The Recap

- Few tasks are more important than identifying and training physician leaders—clinical leaders who will support fellow physicians, help to develop clinical content and workflows, conceive creative ways to gain benefit from the product, and paint a vision of the project that will motivate and excite other clinicians.

- Look for potential physician leaders among those who show an interest in exploring new ways of doing business. The right leader is solution agnostic, not a computer geek—they are interested in improving clinical quality and efficiency, no matter what the tool. Physician leaders also are respected peers, good communicators and, ideally, good teachers.

- Physician leader training can be offered in two, offsite sessions. The first session, in conjunction with project team training, should provide a solid understanding of the system's capabilities. The second training session, for physician leaders alone, should focus on the pros and cons of a variety of solutions to different clinical problems.

- Knowing the common stages of technology adoption will help you to manage users' responses to the EHR. This is especially true of the first stage, the substitutive, which can spawn resistance to the new system if it is not skillfully managed.

- Design your project to move clinicians as rapidly as possible to the second stage of technology adoption, the innovative phase, where most of your success will occur. If you keep at it, before too long you'll realize that you have progressed to the final stage of transformation, where users re-invent the way they provide care and vendors will have to invent new software to keep up with their ideas.

- Use your clinical resources to develop the patient and physician content that is central to physician acceptance of the new system. Don't rely on non-clinical project team members to develop this important element of the EHR.

If You Have Time

- Diffusion of Innovations. Everett M. Rogers. The Free Press; 5th Edition (1995).
- Harvard Business Review on Innovation. Clayton M. Christensen, Michael Overdorf, Ian Macmillan, Rita McGrath, and Stefan Thomke. Harvard Business School Press (2001).

CHAPTER FOUR

Constructing the Project's Foundation: Executive Considerations

In This Chapter
- Define critical success criteria
- Get to know your users' requirements
- Find the right EHR for your needs
- Get the right hardware

To build anything, whether a skyscraper or a new way of structuring health information, the first requirement is a strong foundation. With healthcare organizations, no matter what the project, the real foundation is the executive decision-making process. If the senior team is united in its commitment to a project's success, that project will almost certainly succeed. If they're divided, then the project will often fail.

Again and again, this equation has proven true for health care organizations that implement an electronic health record. Failure almost always results from either a lack of vision at the top or the leadership's inability to convince staff to adopt the vision as their own. In this chapter we'll provide a broad overview of the foundation that your executive team needs to lay in order to establish a successful EHR deployment.

Define Success Criteria

One of the most important elements of a successful EHR implementation is the early identification and constant monitoring of so-called critical success factors. The phrase describes those minimum requirements that the EHR must satisfy in order to assure overall success. For example, in most cases the EHR *must* be capable of submitting charges to a practice management system (PMS). No matter how many fancy, bell-and-whistle applications come with the final EHR, if users can't submit charges then the implementation will have failed. Therefore, compatibility with the PMS is a critical success factor.

It is the executive team's job to assure that the appropriate critical success factors are defined for the implementation. To accomplish this, executives should rely on the input of the soon-to-be physician champions and other end-users, whose first-hand knowledge of everyday workflows assures that no vital system functionality gets overlooked.

Timing is critical. The best strategy is to define critical success factors before you begin shopping for an EHR solution—and then plan your purchase to satisfy the criteria that you've set for yourself. Defining critical success factors early on also helps the project manager prioritize problems that arise during implementation. Any difficult issue that arises at an early stage and does not directly impact a critical success factor should be ignored. Dealing with such peripheral issues at this stage would only eat into the budget without offering much long-term value. Issues that arise in the early stages of implementation should only be addressed then if they directly interfere with a critical success factor. By using the critical success factors as a guide in this way, the project manager can help to keep the project within scope and under budget.

Defining critical success factors is more complex than simply following best practices. Success criteria vary sharply from one organization to the next because the organizations' priorities are different. For instance, an academic organization has very different needs than a large clinic. Most academic organizations think of an EHR, at least in part, as an educational tool. Because students are graded on their performance during patient examinations, a critical success factor of an academic organization's EHR is its ability to support student grading, either directly or indirectly. If indirectly, then the organization must plan to fill in the gaps with additional technology or staffing.

Critical success factors that are common to all EHR implementations and which should never be ignored include strong physician support, dedicated project management, a robust technical infrastructure, a solid training staff, an open-minded project team, and end-user involvement (for more on these success factors, see Chapter Seven). But perhaps the most important of all success factors is executive leadership.

At George Washington University Medical Faculty Associates (MFA) in Washington, D.C., executive leadership was key to the speedy, 30-day implementation of an EHR serving 100 physicians in the summer of 2004. The project's Physician Sponsor, Ryan Bosch, M.D., credits the speed and success of the implementation to the vision of MFA's CEO, Stephen Badger.

"The importance of the CEO and senior management in the success of any electronic health record implementation cannot be understated," says Bosch, who is also an Associate Professor at GWU and Director of MFA's Division of General Internal Medicine. "What stood out in the MFA's implementation versus other implementations I have heard about or participated in was the leadership of the CEO. He was the primary driver of the project. He added accountability at all levels to the project, which was critical to the success of the implementation. Without this accountability, providers tend not to use the system. Especially if there is any perception that this will cause them more work and they do not see the immediate benefit to themselves and their practice."

Know User Requirements and Ensure They're Met

By now you should be familiar with this book's guiding principle - If Doctors Don't Use It, Nothing Else Matters (IDDUINEM). The phrase describes the critical importance of user acceptance—all the time and money put into implementing an EHR will have been wasted if the organization's doctors (not to mention nurses, support staff and department managers) refuse to use it. The focus on understanding and satisfying their requirements should begin with the sales process and continue throughout the stages of project design, testing and support.

As a general rule, to better understand your users' requirements and assure that they're met, plan to include them in each phase of the implementation process. Begin with the sales process. When EHR vendors come to sell their wares, invite a representative team of future users to attend. The team should include at least one physician champion, nurse, support person, etc. Ask the team members to discuss their personal goals for an EHR, as well as their concerns. After you've developed a short-list of vendors, gather the users again and ask them to comment on the products' strengths and weaknesses. Ask them to rate the list of products according to their features (not their cost; focus on issues central to the users' jobs). Then use the resulting ratings to choose the best vendor.

VITALS

The top two reasons why technology projects are impaired and ultimately cancelled are: Incomplete Requirements (13.1%) and Lack of End-User Involvement (12.4%).

Source: The Chaos Report. (1995). www.it-cortex.com/ Stat_Failure_Cause.htm

For instance, if one vendor consistently falls into second place on your users' favorites' list due to a particular feature that most of the users either won't use or just plain dislike, then you should judge that vendor according to the critical success factors. If the troublesome feature would not impact the organization's critical success factors then the product might be worth considering—but only if its cost is significantly (15 percent or more) lower than the users' number one choice—particularly if there is a way to get around the feature(s) of concern. By letting user ratings help with the final decision, you will have saved at least 15 percent on the overall cost of the EHR. That's money that can then be invested in advanced training for lead physicians, or in customizations that are more valuable to the organization

Select the Right EHR for Your Needs

The user rating system is especially valuable in helping wade through the literally hundreds of EHRs, EMRs, CPRs and HISs on the market today. Selecting the right EHR is one of the most confusing and most important decisions you may ever face on the job. Expect to invest some time in finding the right EHR for your organization and ensuring that it fits your needs.

To take a simple example, a fully enabled EHR that is suitable for a 100-physician multi-specialty group may have features that are not required for a 10-doctor cardiology group. That may sound obvious but it illustrates an important point. It's vital that you know enough about your users' requirements to be able to say up front *exactly* what you expect the new EHR to accomplish. It may be that you want a great e-prescribing product, or one that's compatible with the CPOE that interfaces with your primary lab, or a usable solution for your optometrists. The project team will take care of designing the proper workflows, working around deficiencies in the product and determining the best way to transition from paper to the EHR. What you want to define up front is, can this product meet your most critical needs?

A good example comes from Corrections Corporation of America (CCA), the nation's largest owner-operator of private correctional and detention facilities. For its $20 million implementation of an inmate health record, CCA identified several critical needs: an ambulatory EHR that could work in a high-security environment 24 hours a day at 60 locations nationwide and which was capable of supporting security requirements unique to the correctional industry, such as bar-coded identification of inmates. Unfortunately, none of the leading EHR vendors focus on solutions for prisons, so CCA had to find a vendor with the right foundation of security, up-time and cross-location integration and a track-record of providing customized solutions, and then work with them to design their own unique system. Together with the vendor, CCA designed a brand-new component of the EHR—a complete Medication Administration Record built to cope with recidivism, the tendency of inmates to enter and exit the system multiple times over many years. The solution worked very effectively but would never have been possible without clear foresight and planning on the part of CCA.

Because an EHR is quite expensive, you want to be sure to select the system that maximizes value (as outlined in your success criteria) at a minimal cost. How do you determine whether a particular EHR provides good value? One useful but simple analysis is to assign numerical values to each of your success criteria to denote their importance. Say, for instance, that you have three success criteria. You assign Criteria A five points on a scale from one to ten, Criteria B three points, and Criteria C one point. You can then perform the following analysis on each candidate solution:

Candidate Solution Analysis

EHR Solution One:
Cost: $500,000
Criteria met: A and C (6 points)
Result: $500,000/6 = $83,333/Point of Value

EHR Solution Two:
Cost: $900,000
Criteria met: A, B and C (9 points)
Result: $900,000/9 = $100,000/Point of Value

Based on this analysis, Solution One is the better buy because it costs less per point of value, even though it doesn't meet all of your needs. If you can satisfy Criteria B through a customization that costs less than $400,000 (the difference in price between the two solutions), then you should choose Solution One over Solution Two. On the other hand, if the customization of Solution One will cost very nearly $400,000, then paying the extra money for Solution Two may be worth the time and trouble you save.

Get the Right Hardware

Once you've chosen an EHR, the executive team determines the organization's need for support hardware in partnership with the EHR vendor. Be as specific as possible in nailing down the requirements. Provide the vendor with as much detail as possible, including the number of physicians, non-physician clinicians and non-clinician users.

Definition of a rollout strategy will also provide guidance in determining hardware needs. Will you install only e-prescribing and CPOE to start (both have generally low storage requirements and thus lower hardware costs), or will you open with dictation, document/report and a scan solution (which have much higher storage requirements)?

The vendor should be able to provide rough estimates of hardware requirements based on any rollout scenario. But bear in mind that the vendor may only be able to give you industry-wide estimates because hardware requirements vary dramatically based on a number of factors. For example, a specialty group that sees 20 patients per day with an average dictation time of two minutes will require far more storage than a group that sees 30 patients per day with an average dictation time of 30 seconds. Because inaccurate hardware estimates can end up costing you a lot of money, be sure to provide highly detailed specs to the vendor. Remember: No one knows your organization better than you.

In planning your hardware needs, don't forget to consider the future. As a general rule, it's best to seek more capacity than your vendor contract currently calls for. This can help prevent the nightmare scenario of discovering three years after go-live that you have the budget for software upgrades but they can't be successfully implemented because there's no line item for the necessary hardware and support. For a more detailed discussion of hardware, see Chapter Eleven, Technical Considerations: The Critical Role of the IT Department.

The Recap

- The executive decision making process is the foundation of the implementation.
- Define Critical Success Factors before you begin shopping for an EHR. The executive team should define the success factors based on end-user input (remember IDDUINEM).
- Know user requirements and assure they're met.
- Include users in all phases and aspects of the project.
- Carefully analyze vendor solutions to select an EHR that maximizes value for minimal cost.
- Provide highly detailed hardware specs to the vendor. Inaccurate hardware estimates can cost a lot of money.

If You Have Time

- "The CEO's Guide to Health Care Information Systems," by Joseph M. DeLuca and Rebecca Enmark (John Wiley & Sons, Inc.).

- "The Strategic Application of Information Technology in Health Care Organizations," by John P. Glaser (The Jossey-Bass Health Series).

- "Information Systems for Healthcare Management," by Charles J. Austin and Stuart B. Boxerman (Health Administration Press).

- "Health Information Management: Principles and Organization for Health Information Services," edited by Margaret A. Skurka (J-B AHA Press).

CHAPTER FIVE

Measuring Return-on-Investment and Project Success

In This Chapter
- Use ROI to get your project approved
- Learn to identify and measure ROI
- Define financial and non-financial metrics
- Collect and measure baseline data
- Communicate the ROI to stakeholders

A book on implementing an electronic health record would hardly be complete without a discussion of funding for the project. After all, a recent survey by the Medical Records Institute found that the *lack* of funding is the single biggest barrier to implementing an EHR. It need not be so. In this chapter we'll describe how to build a solid business case for getting this project off the drawing table and into the clinic through an analysis of the EHR's return on investment (ROI). Along the way, we'll discuss the many side-benefits of an EHR that are not easily quantified.

How ROI Can Get Your Project Approved

When it comes to making the capital outlay for an EHR, your organization's finance executives will clearly play a critical role. It is their duty to ensure that approved projects are fiscally viable. For most organizations, fiscal viability means maximizing the return to investors. In short, any project that might hurt the financial standing of the organization or keep it from completing its mission will not be approved. Conversely, a project that can offer positive ROI is likely to get a nod from the finance department.

A properly conducted EHR implementation will not only improve the organization's bottom line—by boosting revenues, creating positive returns, and enhancing cash flow—but also improve its ability to deliver non-quantifiable benefits such as improved quality of care and reduced medical errors. The more realistic you are in setting expectations for the EHR, the easier it will be for your organization to transition from the paper past to the digital future. For this reason, it's a good idea to break your analysis down into two broad but related categories: Financial Metrics and Non-Financial Metrics.

Financial Metrics

The most common financial metrics that figure in calculations of ROI come in the form of revenue enhancements, cost reductions, clinical process improvements and reclaimed lost productivity. These categories mirror the promised benefits of the EHR, because an ROI analysis is really nothing more than the process of confirming that the system is delivering its expected benefits. Below are several examples of the financial benefits of an EHR that figure into ROI calculations.

Reductions in Transcription Costs

An EHR allows organizations to realize huge savings by eliminating the need for medical transcription and the personnel who do the transcribing. Many organizations report they are able to reduce their transcription costs by 50 to 90 percent over the first five years of the project, with complete elimination soon thereafter. A case in point: at the Affinity Health Group, a multi-specialty, 27-physician group in Tifton, Georgia, the efficiency of the group's EHR enabled a 50 percent reduction in monthly transcription hours after just one year—from an average 80 hours per month prior to implementation to an average 40 hours per month after implementation. As a result, four part-time transcription positions were eliminated, saving Affinity $28,773 per year. These numbers are not atypical; in fact, other organizations have seen far higher reductions in transcription costs by mandating that physicians use the EHR exclusively for notes.

Cost Savings Through Document Scanning

Implementing document-imaging functionality within an EHR brings multiple financial advantages. For instance, scanned documents are available to physicians via the EHR instantly. That's a significant improvement over the current filing process or transcription process, which often requires up to three weeks for paper documents to make it into a patient's chart. In addition to simplifying access to information, scanning has proven to be more efficient from a resource perspective as the time needed to manage the medical record is significantly reduced.

At Central Utah Clinic (CUC), the largest independent multi-specialty practice in Utah, a study of the effectiveness of scanning versus manual filing determined that CUC's staff was able to file 79 scanned documents in the same amount of time required to file 10 paper documents manually—a nearly 800 percent increase in productivity.

"The time it took for fourteen staff members to do all the loose filing, now only takes three to number, scan, and file to the electronic chart," said Sheri Ford, supervisor of medical records at CUC. "We are able to scan a chart on a walk-in patient in half the time it used to take to pull and deliver the physical chart. We are also free from filing all the little white phone messages, because they are entered electronically. Hallelujah!!"

Besides dramatically reducing the need for staff, scanning also speeds the caregiving process. When every chart is instantly available, providers no longer need to delay appointments while they run around looking for a "lost" chart. Another financial advantage of scanning—medical records rooms and chart storage areas can be emptied and repurposed as additional exam rooms or other revenue-generating space.

VITALS

An EHR implemented in 2004 at George Washington University Medical Faculty Associates in Washington, D.C. saved $254,000 in RN time devoted to chart pulling in the first year alone. Over five years, MFA conservatively estimates it will save more than $6 million in chart-related staffing expenses alone.

Source: GWU/MFA Case Study

Another example of how a scanning solution connected to your EHR will result in ROI returns is in Optical Character Recognition (OCR) processing. This technology can be used to speed up the process of searching Explanation of Benefit (EOB) forms for secondary claims. In the paper world, organizations need to first find the EOB batch (which may be hundreds of pages long), then find the patient, block out or white out the patient data, and connect this data to a HCFA 1500 form. Use of OCR processing allows you to scan in the EOB, and then search and find the pertinent patient information. Why is that important? Because a process that normally takes ten to twenty minutes per claim can be reduced to one to two minutes per claim. That will drastically reduce your backlog of secondary claims awaiting processing and payment.

Increased Charge Dollars, Decreased Charge Lag Time

In the age of falling reimbursements, the ability to manage daily charges is imperative to an organization's survival. Revenue gained from ambulatory patient visits could be enhanced by reducing the amount of missing charges, denied claims and improper ABN notices. Why do so many problems exist in this area? Physicians face a difficult challenge in trying to provide the appropriate documentation for the appropriate level of care. In general, the more highly compensated interactions (and thus codes) require the most stringent documentation. Physicians often lack confidence in their documentation and, as a result, often "down code," choosing the less restrictive (and lower compensated) reimbursement codes, thereby causing significant monetary losses for their practices.

VITALS

George Washington University Medical Faculty Associates saw a one-year gain of nearly $209,000 from more appropriate coding levels due to implementing an EHR. Over five years, MFA estimates better documentation of patient encounters will generate $3.5 million in revenue.

Source: GWU/MFA Case Study

In contrast with the old paper process, an EHR reduces the incidence of under- and over-coding through the use of electronic templates that automatically assign the appropriate billing code, based on the level of care that was documented. When CUC evaluated the impact of their EHR on revenue generated by coding, they found an 11 percent overall increase in appropriate coding following implementation. The resulting reduction in down coding due to the EHR produced an average billable gain of $26 per patient during the study period (2000-2001). When you extrapolate this gain across the entire patient population, it becomes a very compelling ROI.

Reduced Call Backs, Lower Supply Expenses and Staffing Requirements

As most nursing and front desk staff would attest, responding to the large volume of patient phone calls can use up most of the workday. Of course, patient health and satisfaction is why nurses and physicians practice medicine, but significant savings could be realized by answering patients' calls more efficiently. To that end, an EHR enables immediate access to patient data and the generation of tasks among and between the system's users. That functionality can dramatically reduce the number of incomplete messages or illegible post-it notes. Users of the system are able to be more accurate and efficient when handling patient calls and other common office duties.

With the increased efficiency of an EHR comes the ability to better manage resources. Time gained by more effective and efficient access to patient data means employees work smarter and are more productive. As a result, work roles will change, encouraging the reallocation of staff and some attrition—as well as financial savings.

A case in point: at Affinity Health Group, a pre-implementation analysis of workflow efficiencies revealed opportunities for cost-savings in the business office. Affinity's EHR project team discovered that several employees were performing tasks associated with call processing and collections that would prove unnecessary once the EHR was deployed. The new electronic efficiencies allowed the group to outsource its collections department and cut seven full-time equivalent (FTE) positions. These reductions resulted in a net savings (after outsourcing costs) of more than $100,000 annually.

Lastly, it takes a lot of supplies to keep a clinic running in the paper world. Encounter forms, prescription pads, folders, labels, paper, paper, and more paper. Implementing an EHR will do away with the need for many of these supplies and their associated costs.

Repurpose Old Storage Space for Revenue-Generation

Once the EHR is implemented, information that previously filled several rooms with file boxes can now be stored in the space of a few computers. This change allows the organization to free up chart rooms and other storage space, and in some cases repurpose it to revenue generating activities. Costly on-site storage areas can become additional exam or testing rooms. At George Washington University Medical Faculty Associates in Washington,

DC, the implementation of an EHR allowed the organization to scan 4 million pages of documents that previously took up 1,125 square feet of storage space. Since GWU/MFA rents their facility, the savings on rent to store that paper amounted to $472,500 per year (at $35 per square foot).

Non-Financial Metrics

Developing an accurate and fair measure of return on investment requires an examination of a multitude of factors, some of which are less tangible and less easily measured than the financial success factors described above. A thorough examination of the benefits of an EHR should take into consideration, for instance, such complex factors as the potential financial impact of improvements to patient safety and care. While it is difficult to quantify the financial savings that may accrue from enhanced patient safety, recent evidence suggests there is a link.

For example, the EHR's automation of alerts that warn providers of adverse drug reactions or unsafe drug combinations helps to prevent medication errors, which pose a growing problem for the health care industry. According to the 1998 Institute of Medicine (IOM) report, "To Err is Human: Building a Safer Health System," preventable medical errors kill up to 98,000 Americans each year. In examining the IOM's study, the federal Agency for Health Care Research estimated that many of the incidents that resulted in extra hospital days could have been prevented by the implementation of decision-making software and electronic medical records. Reductions in medication errors, in turn, may result in reduced insurance premiums for your organization. Some malpractice insurers are beginning to reduce premiums approximately 5 percent for providers using EHRs, which can mean significant savings.

> **VITALS**
>
> "The impact and expectation of cost-justifying patient safety IT initiatives using a traditional ROI must evolve to focus beyond the financial benefit. It must encompass overall patient safety, patient satisfaction, and employee and physician satisfaction benefit categories."
>
> Source: "Who's Counting Now? ROI for Patient Safety IT Initiatives." L.M. Newell, D. Christensen. *Journal of Healthcare Information Management*

Similarly, an EHR can improve physician compliance with insurance company drug formularies, paving the way for the organization to negotiate better reimbursement rates with its major insurance carriers. Such seemingly non-quantifiable factors can actually have a profound impact on an organization's bottom line not only by reducing malpractice and other insurance premiums but also by encouraging return business from patients.

Other examples of intangible factors that should be considered when calculating ROI include provider satisfaction. Nurses, for instance, can use the EHR to gain instant access to charts with real-time information so they can provide accurate answers to phone questions. An organization's after-hours clinic can access notes from a daytime pediatric visit so nurses can knowledgably advise worried parents. And physicians can join their family for dinner and then, after children are in bed, complete their paperwork over the Internet. These benefits are invaluable to an organization and deliver financial rewards in the form of provider loyalty.

Another EHR capability that's not commonly considered in ROI analysis is the enhanced ability to generate revenue through participation in clinical research studies. Holston Medical Group (HMG), a 71-physician multi-specialty group practice in Kingston, Tennessee, earned more than $1 million from clinical research in 2001 thanks to its EHR. The system can quickly identify patients who are eligible to participate in outcomes-based drug research.

Finally, the timesavings realized from an EHR also can have a positive impact on patient care and your bottom line. By automating routine tasks such as recordkeeping and dictation, an EHR lets physicians spend more time practicing medicine, freeing them to see more patients, which in turn boosts their revenue. And that means ROI.

Collecting and Comparing Metrics

As we have seen, there are a number of areas in which ROI can be quantified by the organization: the time it takes to complete tasks, cost reductions, clinical process improvements, and revenue enhancements. Identifying which of these factors you will use to calculate the EHR's return on investment requires that you first clarify your organization's goals and objectives. Creating a Project Scope document, which is described in Chapter Six, is a good way to clarify goals and objectives. The ROI metrics that you measure should align with the goals and objectives outlined in the scope document. For instance, if one of the organization's goals is to reduce chart-pulling expenses, then you can count on collecting a lot of chart pull numbers to analyze for the ROI.

After identifying the proper metrics, the next step is to establish baseline data against which to measure the EHR's performance. This is the "before and after" scenario—comparing the number of chart pulls before implementation, for instance, to the number of post-implementation chart pulls. In general, aim to measure each of the routine, paper-based clinical and administrative tasks that you expect to be most powerfully affected by the EHR.

The following table can help you decide which baseline data to collect. It provides a list of items commonly collected and measured in calculating ROI for an electronic health record. Please note the associated timeframe for conducting measurements, as some need to be performed exclusively prior to the EHR rollout (marked as "pre" in the table). Additionally, a much more detailed list of ROI measures can be found in Appendix Two.

The EHR's Enhanced Data Mining Capabilities

Gathering detailed metrics is not always easy. In addition to collecting or estimating past performance data for comparison with the present, you will also be required to pull current information directly out of the EHR, once it has been implemented.

Fortunately, the EHR's enhanced data storage and mining capabilities make gathering this sort of information far easier than in the past. Digital information can be gathered from patient charts simply by asking a programmer to spend one hour writing a report query, rather than requiring an analyst to spend days or weeks sifting through the paper charts. The data residing in the EHR can provide answers to a virtually unlimited number of useful questions. For instance, "what's the turn-around time on dictations?" Or, "how many charges were posted without documentation and which ones were they?" The EHR can be used to reveal all diabetes patients with a Hemoglobin A1c value greater than X who have not been seen in three months, or the number who have neither received blood work nor seen their primary care provider in the last six months. The EHR's data mining capabilities also can be used to guide strategic decisions, such as where to build the organization's next cardiology clinic, based on an analysis of the zip codes of your cardiology patients.

What to measure	When to measure
# Chart Pulls: Cost per chart pull	Pre
Chart storage costs	Pre
Chart filing costs	Pre
Percentage of time chart available when patient appointment	Pre
Percentage of time chart available when patient calls	Pre
Paper Costs: paper, copier	Pre/Post
AR days	Pre/Post
Average Charge/ Patient Visit	Pre/Post
Percentage of Denials	Pre/Post
Transcription Costs	Pre/Post
Patient Cycle Time	Pre/Post
Pharmacy Call Backs/ Formulary and hand-writing questions	Pre/Post
Malpractice Rates (inflation and industry adjusted)	Pre/Post
Number of patients seen by provider/ month	Pre/Post

Common ROI Measurements for an Electronic Health Record

Reporting the Good News

As we have seen, there are many ways to show that a well-implemented EHR will save time, make money, and improve the quality of patient care. But those who have only briefly used an EHR may forget these benefits and focus instead on the difficult challenges they faced in deploying and mastering the new system. That's why the final critical element of the ROI equation—after defining, collecting and measuring the data—is to communicate the findings to your users.

This is especially true of non-financial metrics that have a bigger impact on users' day-to-day lives. Examples include a pre- and post-implementation comparison of the number of work hours saved by physicians and the satisfaction of patients (based on survey results). Physicians will want to be reminded of the time they save with the EHR, and the billing department, CIO and CEO will want to see the reduction in collection delays. Once you have the information, therefore, be sure to advertise it.

Measuring the return on investment in individual departments and job functions, as well as organization-wide will help your ROI communication efforts. The more personal the information is, the more impact it will have. A nurse in the Urgent Care clinic, for instance, is likely more interested in hearing about the EHR's impact on patient wait times or medication errors in her department than its role in reducing malpractice premiums for the organization. The point of localizing the ROI is that you can now say to individual departments, "sure, adjusting to the EHR may be tough but here's what it can do for you."

Worth the Journey

The return on investment from an EHR can take many forms. There are gains to be made in operational efficiency, as well as improved patient service. The costs of transcription, paper storage, and chart filing can be dramatically reduced, while improvements in charge coding and quality of care can lead to direct and indirect revenues. Less quantifiable but no less important returns include increased provider and patient satisfaction.

It's an exciting and occasionally challenging road ahead. To make it down this path and come out a leader in patient care, you'll have to jump some hurdles. But just consider the rewards—organization-wide process improvements, better patient care, potentially huge financial gains and an unparalleled view into the minutia of your operations. You can't ask for much better ROI than that.

The Recap

- ROI can help get an EHR project approved by your organization. Positive Net Present Value and Internal Rate of Return values make implementing an EHR a fiscally viable endeavor.

- Collect and measure the metrics that align with your goals and objectives for the EHR. These will typically mirror the promised benefits of the new system.

- Set realistic ROI goals. Base expectations on industry standards and define what project success means at your organization.

- Save on Transcription costs. Implementing an EHR can dramatically decrease expenses related to transcription services as the system offers alternative methods for capturing this data.

- Save on the cost of supplies. Remove the cost associated with preparing and maintaining patient medical charts, as well as encounter forms and prescription pads.

- Increase charge dollars. EHRs help physicians provide the documentation necessary to improve proper coding, driving revenue gains.

- Reduce FTE numbers and reclaim lost hours. Efficiencies garnered from the EHR will allow personnel to be reallocated to other tasks and may eliminate the need for certain positions.

- Repurpose old chart rooms to revenue generating activities. Costly on-site storage areas can become additional exam or testing rooms.

- Lower the costs related to malpractice insurance by improving patient safety.

If You Have Time

- Fifth Annual Medical Records Institute's Survey of Electronic Health Record Trends and Usage (2003). http://www.medrecinst.com/pages/libArticle.asp?id=41.

- A Multi-method Quality Improvement Intervention To Improve Preventive Cardiovascular Care. S. Ornstein. Annals of Internal Medicine (October 5, 2004).

- Putting A Clamp on Medical Mishaps. M. McGee. Healthcare Financial Management (January 2002).

- Rapid Implementation of an EMR, a presentation by Chris Madden, M.D., at the Clinical Computing Executive Summit (August 25, 2004).

- The Economic Effect of Implementing an EMR in an Outpatient Clinical Setting. S. Barlow, J. Johnson, J. Steck. Journal of Healthcare Information Management (Winter 2004).

- Electronic Medical Record Sets Group Apart as e-Pioneers and Delivers Powerful Advantages. Microsoft Customer Solution: Healthcare Industry (September 2002).

CHAPTER SIX

Planning, Management and Control: The Project Manager's Role

In This Chapter
- Prepare the foundation for implementing the EHR
- Design the EHR project plan
- Build and test the new system
- Train the end-users
- Go live with the new system

In many respects, an EHR implementation is just like any other IT project. You discover what needs to be done, plan how to accomplish it, do the work, measure the results and bring the project to a close. But there's one critical difference: if the EHR project fails, the organization's core mission of patient care will be compromised. With the stakes so high, it's a good idea to plan in advance.

This chapter will set the foundation for a successful implementation by introducing the tools and methods of traditional project planning and management. We'll outline typical project activities and lead you through the development of the project scope and formalize a project plan. Finally, we'll show you how to manage and control the EHR implementation by following best practices.

What Exactly Is Project Management?

According to the Project Management Institute, a project is "a temporary endeavor undertaken to create a unique product or service." Implementing an EHR at a medical clinic or facility would certainly qualify as creating a unique service. An electronic health record is intended to dramatically improve the quality of care and the efficiency of the medical staff while saving the organization money.

Heading up this ambitious effort is the Project Manager, who is responsible for identifying the implementation project's objectives, assembling a plan for achieving them, and carrying out the execution of that plan.

The Project Manger must be an experienced planner and leader—someone who remains calm and focused even in the middle of a crisis, and who is able to quickly adjust to changing conditions. The position is so critical to the implementation's success that it should ideally be filled only by a person with previous EHR experience. However, if a Project Manager with EHR experience is not available, then the next best choice would be one with experience implementing enterprise applications. Less desirable in this position is an existing line manager or team lead, since these managers are accustomed to tasks that are far more repetitive and short-term than the tasks associated with a months'-long project. It's also a bad idea to view the management of an EHR implementation as a growth opportunity for a promising but inexperienced employee. Why take chances on a project that will directly impact the mission-critical functions and services of your organization?

The Project Manager's blueprint for the implementation is called the "project management methodology." Several different management methodologies are available on the market, including the Microsoft Solution Framework, Franklin Covey's Project Management Approach, the Rational Unified Process, and others. All of them address the same three core-planning processes: *design*, *develop* and *deliver*. The 3-D™ methodology borrows from several different management styles, industry best practices, and client experiences. If your EHR vendor offers such a methodology, you would be wise to review it and seriously consider using all or part of it to guide your EHR implementation. An experienced Project Manager also will be able to guide you through this process.

In this chapter we'll describe a generic project management methodology consisting of five essential processes: Prepare, Design, Develop, Deliver and Advance. The diagram on the following page describes the methodology and its milestones. You can refer back to the diagram in the discussion that follows.

	I.Prepare	II. Design	III. Develop	IV. Deliver	V. Advance
STEPS	Project Introduction	Develop Project Scope & Control Plan	Execute the Project Plan	Train Users	Quality Control
	Gather Requirements	Conduct a Risk Assessment	Build the System	Scope Change Control	Project Evaluation
	Define Objectives	Develop a Communication Plan	Test the System	Go-Live	Support Transition
	Define Responsibilities	Develop Change Management Plan	Develop Training Materials	Report Progress	Report Results
	Determine Resource Needs	Develop the Project Plan	Develop Go-Live Planning	Executive Status Review	Executive Status Review
	Determine System Needs	Develop Training Plans	Scope Change Control		
	Report Progress	Report Progress	Report Progress		
	Executive Status Review	Executive Status Review	Executive Status Review		

Basic Project Management Methodology

Project Management Methodology: Prepare, Design, Develop, Deliver, and Advance

The first three processes in the project management methodology (prepare, design and develop) share the underlying theme of identifying needs and planning for their development. This emphasis on identifying project needs and planning the execution of the project ahead of time is considered a best practice for a couple of reasons. First, rather obviously, the more critical needs you identify in advance, the easier it will be to plan to satisfy those needs. Second, good planning keeps the team from wasting time on problems they should have foreseen in the planning stage.

The Prepare Process

The Prepare process begins with introducing the project to the organization and declaring a deadline. After the introduction, the remaining milestones can be completed in virtually any order. For example, if you're waiting for confirmation of a key consultation or meeting, and it's known that a Virtual Private Network (VPN) connection needs to be installed for later development work, then by all means stop waiting around and get the VPN hook up out of the way. In short, do whatever can be done to get the project moving and building momentum.

Bear in mind that the Prepare process will set the tone for the entire implementation. Tone and mood are important because implementing an EHR requires that significant process changes be made to everyday clinical tasks. Change management plans may be part of the Design process, but the seed is planted during the Prepare phase.

Requirements Gathering

Referring back to the methodology diagram, the "gathering requirements" milestone is achieved by identifying the organizations' needs and finding the proper EHR solution to meet those needs. Don't be fooled into accepting the standard explanation that requirements gathering is simply about collecting information from users. This important process is also the opportune time to identify what the various EHR solutions under consideration may require of the medical organization in terms of hardware, software, operating systems, security access, staff, and interfaces with other systems. The earlier these requirements are recognized, the easier it will be to accomplish them. For example, it is far more difficult to add major new features to the EHR's functionality after the implementation has progressed than it is at the start.

Define Project Objectives and Staffing Requirements

The next milestone is defining the project's objectives. Without knowing the objectives that the project was designed to accomplish, you cannot evaluate the success or failure of the implementation. At this point, the objectives are no more than desired outcomes expressed by project sponsors and senior management. Later on, they will be refined into what is to be accomplished, also known as the project scope. (For more on defining objectives, see the discussion below on the project scope document).

Once the objectives are clearly outlined, the Project Manager can use them to determine the project's staffing needs and assign responsibilities. Staffing an EHR implementation is a dynamic process because the new system impacts so many other existing systems. As a result, help is needed from a variety of sources—new employees hired specifically for the project; current employees borrowed from other organizational areas; and outside vendors. Project Managers with EHR implementation experience can be quite helpful in this area because they are accustomed to juggling the numerous resources and deliverables involved in such a high-demand project. (For detailed suggestions on staffing the Project Team, see Chapter Seven, Building and Managing Effective Project Teams).

Determine System Needs

This next milestone requires you to take a hard look at the organizations' existing IT infrastructure (for more on this topic, see Chapter Eleven, The Right Tool for the Job). Work with your IT staff to answer some common sense questions about the implementation. Will any of the systems need to be upgraded? Will adding the new system degrade overall network performance? Will remote users be able to efficiently access the EHR? Can the new system be built using older hardware currently in use by another mission-critical system, or will it require all-new hardware?

Understanding the existing infrastructure plays a big role in developing the project budget and schedule because new hardware can significantly impact the project's cost and timeline. A common mistake in IT projects is to delay consideration of infrastructure needs until the Design or Development process. But waiting until that late date to identify infrastructure changes increases the likelihood of a slip or an additional budget request.

The Prepare process is usually determined to be complete by an executive status review involving the project's major stakeholders. Periodic reviews may be necessary from time to time.

The Design Process

The objectives of the Design process are to:

1. Identify the target deliverables
2. Assemble a plan for achieving the deliverables
3. Identify any risks that may hamper the team's ability to achieve the deliverables
4. Determine how to respond to changes and deviations from the plan
5. Determine the proper channels and methods for communicating the plan, deliverables, updates, issues, and contingencies

Write the Scope Document

The Design process begins with the development of the project scope and the implementation plan. Every Project Manager should live by these two documents, which together define the "who, what, where, when, why and how" of the project. Specifically, the scope defines exactly *what* needs to get done and *why*. The implementation plan is the roadmap for achieving the scope, including *who* will be involved, *where* and *how* it will be implemented, and *when* completion is expected.

The scope is where it all begins. For a project to succeed, the scope must be clearly stated, easily understood, and broadly agreed upon. If the scope is too vague, it's open to interpretation and invites others to include their pet projects in the project. If it's too strict, then important changes that could improve the EHR will be rejected for being unaligned with the scope. As a result, the project will deliver less value to the organization.

So what's the secret to finding the middle ground between vagueness and exactitude? One suggestion is to ask everyone involved in the project what they would ideally like to achieve with the implementation, and then figure out how much of what they want is possible. If a goal inflates the budget, lengthens the timeline or is just plain impractical, then it is removed from the scope. Also cut anything that lacks a simple, clear-cut case for its inclusion. Following this culling process, any goal that's left is worth pursuing and should be included in the project.

After producing a first draft of the project scope document, it's a good idea to get other project managers or colleagues to review it. They will be able to spot any obvious openings in the tight language of the scope that could be subject to interpretation. Next, run the scope by the Executive Sponsor and the Physician Sponsor to assure it fulfills their vision for the project. If one of the sponsors insists on including additional objectives in the scope, then the Project Manager must be prepared to explain how the proposed change would affect the original mission, the project budget and timeline. Such a response will either encourage the sponsor to withdraw their request, or persuade them to champion the change by seeking the necessary additional resources from senior management. Either way, the Project Manager's aim should be to clearly define the project scope without endangering the health of the project early on.

Finally, the scope should be reviewed again to ensure that it is precise enough to allow the Project Manager to swiftly decide whether a proposed change to the project has merit or not. Run through a few hypothetical scenarios to see whether the scope would serve as a good measuring tool in those situations. If it's not precise enough, then keep working at it. If it is, then you're ready to present it and get it approved.

Prepare the Implementation Plan

Once you get sign-off on the scope document, it's time to begin writing the EHR implementation plan. The implementation plan can't be finalized until the scope is approved because it's the blueprint for accomplishing the objectives set out in the scope. If the scope gives priority to specific EHR functionalities, then this affects *how* the system is implemented. If the scope mentions which existing systems will interface with the EHR, then that defines *who* will be working on the project. Ditto for *where* and *when* the project will be implemented.

The Work Breakdown Structure

To help assemble the implementation plan and determine how the scope will be achieved, a good tool and a project management best practice is a Work Breakdown Structure (WBS). A WBS lists all the tasks to be accomplished for the project, groups them into logical clusters, and places them in the order they need to be performed.

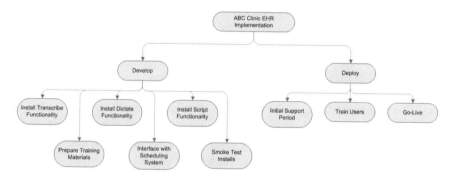

Sample Work Breakdown Structure

To create the WBS, identify the tasks associated with each objective outlined in the project scope, and then map them according to the physical location of the work (i.e., General Medicine, Urgent Care, Clinic A, etc.) and its priority on a timeline. Note that, at this time, only the priority of the tasks is important. Later on, while constructing the Network Diagram, the timing for each task will be mapped out.

The WBS is a relatively simple process that makes it easier to determine the location and timing of project tasks. For example, if it's known that Clinic #1 (out of five) requires a new data line with greater bandwidth to accommodate the EHR, then installing that data line is a task that should be added to the WBS Under Clinic #1 tasks. However, if it's known that all five clinics need to be evaluated for a new data line, then the specific location of the task doesn't matter—it has to happen across the board. In that case, installing a new data line is added to the WBS as one task that needs to be completed at all locations.

After the WBS has been mapped out, you can use it to help determine who will be asked to achieve the project goals outlined in the project plan. Will regular employees be used? Offshore contractors? Local contractors? A third-party vendor or supplier? The answer will be different for each task but it's vital that you get the answers early because the type of resource that is used will figure heavily in estimating the project timeline. Simply estimating the number of person-hours needed to complete each individual task in the WBS can create a high-level estimation of the duration of the project. Roll these individual time estimates up to their parent levels in the WBS and you'll have an initial idea of how the project will be staffed, what steps need to be taken when, and an estimated completion date. Finally, the Project Manager should refine the estimates and incorporate more realistic implementation scenarios into the project structure.

The Network Diagram

A second useful tool and project management best practice that can be created after the WBS has been completed is a network diagram. A network diagram uses the group labels for WBS tasks to construct a matrix based on dependency, constraints, and estimated completion time.

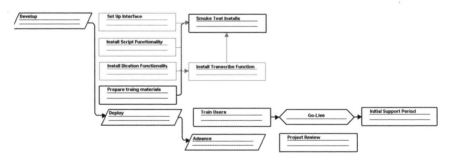

Sample Network Diagram

When moving the labels from the WBS to the network diagram, all repetitive groupings or tasks need to be broken out into individual listings. For example, if the task of evaluating data lines is listed once on the WBS for all five clinics, then it needs to be listed on the network diagram five times (e.g., "Evaluate Data Line—Clinic #1", "Evaluate Data Line—Clinic #2", etc.).

Breaking out the WBS labels helps to identify the "critical path," or the shortest route to achieving the project scope objectives for the implementation. On Figure 6.2 the boxes with the red outline and the white backgrounds represent the critical path. Determining the critical path is a complex process that considers numerous factors, including resources needed for each task, delays in other projects due to staff reassignments, other changes in staffing, holiday seasons, and IT department freeze periods. During the development process, if any of these factors unexpectedly change, the critical path may be impacted and even dramatically shifted.

Unfortunately, calculating a critical path or making adjustments to it based on project progress is beyond the scope of this chapter. Please see the Additional Information section at the end of the chapter for further reading on the topic.

The Project Schedule

Once the network diagram is complete, it should give the Project Manager a clear picture of the implementation's "who, what, where, when, why and how." Now the Project Manager can use the diagram to create a project schedule. The schedule is primarily used for tracking and measuring the implementation's progress, but it can also be used as a planning tool.

To build the project schedule, take the tasks that you added to the network diagram—along with their estimated durations, their dependencies, and the resources assigned to them—and assign them specific start and end dates. The schedule usually includes a graphical representation of the timeline (the right side of Figure 6.3) that names the person responsible for completing the task. Also factored in at this time are vacations, holidays, and other calendar-related issues. During the Design process the project schedule is used for planning the start-date of tasks and what resources need to be on hand to accomplish them. The schedule will be used again during the Development and Deliver stages to track project progress and coordinate resources.

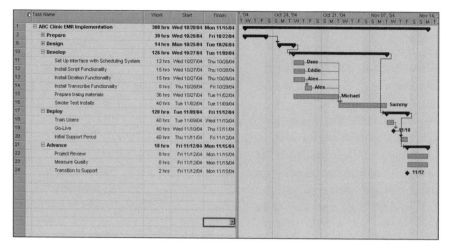

Sample Project Schedule

Assessing Risks and Planning for Change

After the project scope and project plan have been assembled, it's time to identify any possible threats that could jeopardize the project's objectives. This is the point in the project at which risk assessment and change-control planning come into play.

The risk assessment identifies all potential threats to the project, evaluates the probability of each threat, and gauges their potential impacts on the project. The risks are actually quite real and, if realized, could endanger the success of the implementation. For example, providers and clinical staff could decide that the new system's functionality isn't acceptable, or that the EHR delivers poor performance on a mission-critical task or process. The project team could underestimate the implementation's impact on the organization. Government regulation or new legislation could dramatically alter the technical or procedural requirements of an EHR. Or the organization could have trouble bringing enough users live on the EHR prior to a particularly busy season.

Risks can be rated on a "threat scale," ranging from high to low depending on their probability and potential severity. The higher the risk, the greater the threat; the lower the risk, the lower the threat. You can determine the severity of a risk by considering objective as well as subjective information. For instance, if the project will introduce tablet PCs to providers, then the subjective information you might consider in determining the risk level associated with the move could include the providers' general willingness to change, their willingness to learn new computer skills, and the support staff's personal feelings regarding the tablets. Objective factors to consider in assessing the risk of the tablet PC introduction include known issues reported by the manufacturer, product recalls, and product availability. By considering both subjective and objective factors, you should be able to deduce the probability of a risk occurring and its severity.

After the project risks have been identified and their severity evaluated, prepare an informal contingency plan for minimizing each risk. You will have to monitor risks throughout the project, as long as they pose a threat. Don't be surprised if new, unexpected risks appear as the project proceeds. These risks, too, will have to be assessed and monitored.

Developing a Change Management Plan

Risks sometimes lead to suggestions that the implementation plan should be changed. Other suggestions for changes can come from managers, administrators, providers, clinical staff, or the Project Team itself. Changes to the project may also be required by unexpected organizational adjustments, acquisitions, or government regulations. But before you actually agree to change the project plan, a change-control process should be prepared and agreed upon.

The change management process kicks in when someone involved with the project submits a change request for consideration by the Project Manager. The Project Manager then conducts an impact analysis using the project scope, the network diagram, and the project schedule. The first question should always be, "does the request fall within the scope of the project?" If it falls outside of the scope and would threaten the implementation's success, then the request should be denied or added to a list of potential future upgrades. If the request falls within the scope, and/or presents a danger if *not* implemented, then it graduates to the next consideration: "How would the request impact the critical path and project schedule?"

At this point the change request should be run through the WBS process, added to the network diagram and compared against the project schedule. The Project Manager should also evaluate how adding the request to the project plan will impact the critical path and scheduling commitments. Not only change requests but also anything that could have an impact on the project's deliverables must be tested against the critical path and the schedule. If it is found that the change would shorten, shift, or lengthen the critical path or schedule, the item should be taken under careful consideration. The Project Manager must eventually approve, deny, or delay the request for a future release or upgrade. All parties involved with the request should be informed of the decision and agree to move forward in achieving the project's deliverables, regardless of the outcome.

The Communication Plan

To maintain the project's momentum and the morale of everyone involved, it's important to provide regular progress reports, and to communicate decisions and the status of any risk items. This information must be communicated in a professional manner by the appropriate sources to prevent gossip and inaccuracies from harming the project.

The communication plan (see Appendix Three for a sample plan) outlines who on the Project Team will communicate what information to whom and under what conditions. The plan is a critical part of any EHR implementation not only for the reasons already outlined but also because it helps to ensure that no one is left out of important announcements. Missed communications can snowball and may eventually lead to improper development, missed deliverables, or outright confusion. Such misunderstandings are magnified when third-party vendors and outside resources are part of the mix. Think of the vendors and contractors as members of the team, the same as internal resources, and include them in the communications plan.

A.J. Schuler, PsyD, an expert in leadership solutions and change management, advises that to win people's commitment for change, you must engage their interest on both a rational level and an emotional level. You can take Schuler's advice to heart by assuring that your communication plan addresses the emotional impact of the coming change as well as the facts behind it. Areas to cover in the plan include:

* Organizational Objectives: Explain the organization's overall objectives for the EHR. What does the organization hope to accomplish, and what are its deadlines for accomplishing it? How will success be measured and communicated?

- The organization's responsibilities and expectations: Explain the organization's responsibility for helping users prepare for change through education and ongoing support.

- The users' responsibilities and expectations: Explain what is expected of the users regarding time devoted to training and practice, and their responsibility for knowledge retention and evaluation.

- Personal Objectives: What's in it for me? Why would I, the user, want or need to use this system?

As you formulate the communication plan, remember that successful communication is not a one-time event—it's a continuous process. The organization should measure and communicate progress on the EHR implementation on a regular basis. Consistent, timely communication helps maintain user support for the EHR. Conversely, inconsistent, or untimely information that's unskillfully presented can endanger user support for the implementation. And don't forget to regularly review your communication plan to assure your organization is sticking to it. When people are kept in the dark, they're more likely to create misinformation that's passed along through back channels or gossip.

Be especially careful to include the clinical leadership and super users at each clinic in the communications plan. Their pivotal role in building support for the EHR among physicians makes it all the more critical for the Core Project Team to maintain frequent communication with them. As we will discuss in Chapter Eight, the plan should aim to keep them in the loop on all aspects of the project's progress.

Developing the communications plan may not be the most glorious part of being a Project Manager but remember—it takes well-informed people to make informed decisions.

The Develop Process

By this point in the implementation, the Prepare and Design stages have been completed and "go fever" is starting to set in. That's a good sign that it's time to start focusing on the Develop process—the execution of all the preparations and designs you've worked so hard to put in place. Project management emphasis now begins to shift away from planning and towards keeping things on track.

Building and Testing the System

The major milestones of the Develop process are the building and testing of the system. Unless you complete these two milestones, the project will not be able to continue. For a detailed discussion of the building and testing stages of implementation, see Chapter Ten, Assuring Quality and Operational Readiness). Briefly, building the system involves a myriad of tasks, including setting up user access, setting system preferences, and tying into existing or external systems. System testing is a bit like the old Samsonite commercials on TV, in which a gorilla is made a gift of a new suitcase. System testing is akin to the gorilla's bashing of the suitcase; it attempts to uncover lapses in the system, to break a process flow or piece of functionality. It's far better to uncover and fix a serious fault early than to risk it surfacing after go-live.

The Project Manager's role during the Develop process is largely to focus on tracking the project's progress, mediating issues, and putting out fires. The PM also is more likely to be confronted by change requests during this stage as more new requirements are identified. For example, if system testing reveals that a supervising signature is required for approving specific lab tests or prescriptions, then some workflow settings and permissions will need to be changed. Some of the most commonly missed system requirements include permission settings, entering provider DEA and state licensing information, office-visit note structuring, associating lab tests with the proper result-able items, backfilling vital patient information into the new system, proper printing destinations for documents, lab or script vendor requirements, and vital networking or infrastructure needs. If you experience low numbers of scope change requests and few unrealized requirements, then it's clear you did a good job preparing for and designing the project.

Depending on the skill and experience of the Project Manager, they may be asked to gather and document detailed requirements or specific needs of the medical staff. The detailed requirements let the Project Team know how the system needs to be configured and what subjects need to be covered during user training. For example, prior to the implementation of the EHR, the process of refilling prescriptions involves several steps: 1) receiving a refill request, 2) pulling a patient chart, 3) routing the chart and the request to a clinical staff member, 4) confirming validation of the request by the provider, and 5) receiving the final decision. After the EHR is implemented, this process will change. The Project Manager's job is to align the requirements above with the capabilities of the new system, thus ensuring that when a refill request is received, the provider is electronically notified to review that patient's medical information in the system and send any approved scripts to the pharmacy via the EHR.

Detailed requirements also help to reveal the type of learning materials that will be needed for user training. In the refill example above, for instance, it's obvious that clinical staff will have to learn how to task providers with refill requests and providers will need to learn how to write scripts using the EHR. Procedure manuals or cheat sheets might be created to assist in training users to do this. It's important to get an early jump on the development of training materials, just in case the Project Team runs into any content or printing problems. It would be a shame to jeopardize the project's success by failing to provide enough training materials for the users. Remember, the users will only have their training materials to fall back on during those fun, first days of go-live. Make sure the materials are easy to follow, but not so easy that they fail to provide the necessary information for each situation.

The Deliver Process

"Go fever" is at an all time pitch now. It's time to light this candle, put your money where your mouth is, lay it all on the line, and ... well, you get the picture. The team has gathered the requirements, planned the training lessons, prepared the training materials, scheduled the users for training, and planned the go-live. By now, the Project Team and the Project Manager should have wrapped up their planning activities and begun to focus one-hundred percent on implementation and support.

In essence, it is during the Deliver process that the team finishes up the remaining planned tasks and goes live with the new system. This involves training all the users, turning them loose in the live system, and assisting them with any questions or problems. If the Project Manager has done their job correctly, they should have some time available to help out with assisting the implementation team, answering user questions, and dealing with minor issues that pop up. Up until now, the major responsibilities of the Project Manager have been to assemble the project plan, make sure that the implementation team is following the plan, resolve issues that develop along the way, and track the team's progress. During the Deliver process, it's a good idea for the Project Manager to conduct a final go-live prep meeting and then either assist end users or research reported missed requirements.

The Advance Process

At long last, the EHR system has been implemented and the users are up and running on it. Now it's time to release the remaining resources and shift the remaining EHR IT team from an implementation mode to a support mode. Accomplishing this means verifying that the system is stable, running efficiently, and meeting the needs of the providers and clinical staff. The Project Manager should now verify and communicate to the project sponsors the successes and/or failures of meeting the provider's needs and the project's objectives.

Going forward, quality control will be the primary emphasis for the EHR IT team. They'll focus on recovering user errors, keeping the system running efficiently, dealing with system bugs, helping the users to incorporate new needs into the system, and installing upgrades.

Project Evaluation

The final task for the Project Manager should be to conduct a project evaluation meeting. At this gathering, all of the project control data is presented to the Project Team and sponsors for review. This data is important because its findings can be used in future EHR implementations and other future projects.

If additional functionality needs to be implemented or deployed, or if a there are outstanding change requests waiting in line to be implemented, then another pass through the Development cycle may be required. Rather than wrapping up the project at this time, the Project Manager may need to partially transfer some of the effort to a support mode and continue leading the implementation.

Keeping the Project Under Control

Keeping any project under control is always a priority, and this book should help in that regard. But don't forget that complete control is a dangerous illusion. Influences outside of your control include unexpected personnel changes, illnesses, re-organizations, government mandates, and uncountable other factors up to and including acts of God (tsunamis, earthquakes, etc.). On top of everything else, in the medical world the Project Manager has to be prepared to confront the realities of dynamic patient loads and staff being pulled away at any given moment to respond to an emergency.

How can you be expected to plan for such events and still keep the project under control? The unfortunate truth is that you will probably never be fully prepared to handle every obstacle that might potentially derail the project. But you can help reduce the impact of an unexpected event by working to *influence* the situation rather than *controlling* it.

Influencing the outcome of a situation is far easier than trying to control the outcome. For starters, influencing is more dynamic in nature, while controlling is static and procedural. Influencing leaves room for flexibility and creativity. Controlling leaves room only for more controls. The intention behind good EHR project management is simply this: to be guided by the project's objectives; to plan for as many contingencies as possible; to reduce as many risks as possible; and to keep the team's morale up so they're better able to respond effectively to unexpected, troubling events when they occur.

The Recap

- New EHR = Big change, impacting core workflow processes. Need to analyze and design- Need to have an experienced EHR Project Manager (PM), or at the very least an experienced IT PM (would you want any less when implementing a mission critical system?).
- Determine objectives and scope up front and stick to them throughout the project.
- Get good requirements. Map processes. Create test plans. All three help to insure you get it right!
- Risk Analysis—Do it when preparing the project plan, determine action plans for each risk, and maintain throughout the project.
- Work Breakdown Structure, Network Diagrams, and Project Schedules. Create and maintain to keep project on track.
- Establish a clear communication plan for all so issues are resolved quickly and appropriately.
- PM also means Planning and Measuring. Plan as much as possible in order to avoid surprises and measure how well the planning was done (so it can be used for future projects).

If You Have the Time

- The Project Management Institute (www.pmi.org).
- The Rational Unified Process
  (www.306.ibm.com/software/awdtools/rup/).
- The Microsoft Solution Framework (www.microsoft.com/technet/itsolutions/techguide/msf/default.mspx).
- FranklinCovey (www.franklincovey.com).
- Tech Republic IT Management (http://techrepublic.com.com/1200-22-5349192.html).

CHAPTER SEVEN

Building and Managing Effective Project Teams

In This Chapter
- Elements of a successful project team
- Design the project team structure
- Build project team governance
- Assemble, launch and develop your teams
- Monitor and evaluate team progress

To ensure that the work of implementation and support is in good hands, leadership should give careful consideration to the organizational roles required for success and how best to staff and manage those roles. In this chapter we present a roadmap to building a successful project team and leading it through the dynamic process of implementing the EHR.

The roadmap can be summarized as a ten-step process:

1. Understand the components of successful EHR project teams
2. Build the right roles for the right people
3. Determine how much (and where) to invest in the project team
4. Finalize the structure of your teams
5. Establish a system of project governance
6. Assemble your teams
7. Launch your teams
8. Develop your teams
9. Monitor, evaluate and facilitate team progress

10. Maintain a motivational team environment

For each step we'll cover the challenges you may face and make recommendations that will help you overcome them on your way to staffing a successful EHR program.

Step One: Understand the Components of Successful EHR Project Teams

Experience has shown that the most successful EHR implementations are those that adopt a project team structure made up of five essential components: Executive and physician leadership; the core project team; clinical leadership; the IS support team; and third-party vendors (the EHR vendor, labs, radiology, pharmacies, etc.). Each component has unique responsibilities that can only be fulfilled by its members. Together, all five contribute to one cohesive, smoothly functioning project team.

It's best to begin developing each of the five project components before selecting an EHR vendor. This is true for three reasons. First, by participating in the evaluation of different EHR solutions, the team members from all five groups gain insight into the key goals and objectives of the new system. That, in turn, will help them make the right decisions from the very beginning. Second, forming the project teams early provides them with the time they need to get their bearings and develop into cohesive, high-performing teams—a prerequisite to avoiding costly delays and poor decisions during the implementation.

VITALS

Building effective project teams requires more than simply matching the right people to the right roles. Three other elements are key to ensuring the long-term success of your vision: Providing adequate resources to your teams; backing the teams with the full weight of executive support; and performing advanced planning for a smooth transition to support services once the implementation is complete.

Finally, effective change management requires early and regular communication with key stakeholders. Many of these stakeholders will serve as the overall project's executive or physician leaders or as local leaders within clinics. By involving them early and also keeping others informed, you can boost awareness of the impending opportunity for change and encourage buy-in and participation.

Key EHR Project Team Roles

Following is a breakdown of the roles within each component of a successful project team, including a summary of each group's responsibilities.

Executive/Physician Leadership

> **Executive Sponsor**
> **Physician Sponsor(s)**
> **Influential Physician Leadership**
> **EHR Steering Committee**

The project's leadership usually consists of an Executive Sponsor and a primary Physician Sponsor (often joined by additional physicians and executives who play secondary roles). These leaders are involved in the definition of expected outcomes and boundaries for change, as well as ensuring that organizational support is strong for the other components of the project team structure. The Executive Sponsor, in particular, is responsible for monitoring and facilitating the effectiveness of all the project teams and thus the progress of the entire project. The executive in this key role should have sufficient direct decision-making authority for the majority of weekly issues that will typically be passed on by the Project Manager.

The Executive Sponsor and the physician leadership should form an EHR Steering Committee with operational leaders across the organization to ensure the project's goals and priorities are sufficiently aligned with the organization's strategic direction. The Steering Committee will serve as the primary approval forum for new EHR-driven clinical and operational processes and procedures, and will be the ultimate decision-making authority when consensus fails. Larger, multi-specialty organizations will often separate the clinical arm of this decision making body into a separate Clinical Advisory Board. In this scenario, the EHR Steering Committee will include a much smaller representation from the clinical community and will focus more on project governance issues (for more on governance, see Step Five). The separate Clinical Advisory Board is then responsible for swift decisions on clinical design matters, which minimizes the time of all representative physicians and nursing staff.

The executive leaders, physician leaders and EHR Steering Committee executives will be responsible for final approval of system design and configuration as well as for promoting and influencing utilization of the EHR within their own departments or clinics.

Core Project Team

> **Project Manager**
> **Clinical and operational specialists**
> **Business/ancillary systems' management**
> **Training Coordinator/trainer(s)**
> **Integration and conversion analyst(s)**
> **IS lead**

The Core Project Team is a small but diverse group that is built for speed and effectiveness. This team should be involved from the project's inception. Once the project begins, the members of the Core Project Team will be intimately involved in all day-to-day operations of the implementation and must collectively possess a clear understanding of current clinical and office workflows and future user needs. The Core Project Team will be held accountable for project management, data gathering, design decisions, system configuration, interface design, integration testing, end-user training and facilitating system acceptance with clinical users. When the work in these areas is not done directly by the Core Project Team, they will be responsible for coordinating organizational resources to accomplish these tasks.

For deployment projects in more complex organizations (multi-specialty, academic settings or organizations with more than 200 providers), it's common to branch the Core Project Team into multiple sub-teams, especially when the EHR is implemented in a phased rollout to end-users. For example, one team may be established to focus on work associated with the initial implementation of modules. This team would work with showcase clinics to design new processes and oversee integration with other systems, configure and validate the EHR, train users and support the go-live events for the first modules of the phased system. Once the showcase clinics have gone live with the first EHR modules, a second project team would be responsible for working with each subsequent clinic and/or specialty to refine and validate the system configuration, train end-users and support each live event. This dual approach can be a more effective means of managing and supporting change within a larger organization.

Clinic Leadership

The local clinic leadership, sometimes referred to as an advance team, includes managers, supervisors, influential physicians and other key staff members who are energized learners eager to share their knowledge with the clinic's end users. These leaders will assist in the management of change at each location or clinic through their involvement in the review of the system design and validation of the system configuration. The Project Manager will rely on their local knowledge to determine the project's timing, to uncover potential risks and identify key influencers in their clinics.

Soliciting the participation of this small group of physicians and support staff is a powerful mechanism to affect change at the clinic level. The clinic leadership should be required to participate in design review sessions in which they'll validate (or invalidate) and refine the initial design and workflow recommendations made by the Core Project Team (prior to configuration of the EHR). Once the final workflows are configured, these same people will assess the new clinical workflows during simulation testing to ensure that everything works properly prior to live use.

VITALS: KEYS TO A SUCCESSFUL PHYSICIAN CHAMPION:

- Respected by peers
- Flexible and accepting of new processes and change
- Basic understanding of software and technology
- Ability to ease concerns and help peers with transition to technology
- Convince peers that the value is worth the effort, focusing on quality of care
- Have "thick skin" and willing to stay the course
- Recognize that success requires a lot of work, but is worth it in the long run

It's typical for the clinical leadership team to be designated "super users," thanks to their early and in-depth exposure to the EHR. The clinic's other physicians and local end-users can leverage the super users' advanced knowledge and proficiency early in the adoption process. As mentioned in the previous chapter, their pivotal role makes it all the more critical for the Core Project Team to maintain frequent communication with them through a change-management communication plan. This plan should facilitate communication in both directions. From a top-down perspective, the plan should facilitate education of the leadership and super users at each clinic and keep them in the loop on the project's progress. At the same time, the Core Project Team and Executive Sponsor will want to solicit feedback from the clinics before, during and after local implementation.

> ## VITALS
>
> **The Super Users' mastery of the EHR is vital to speeding the system's implementation. Because their heavy responsibility comes on top of their current jobs, many organizations reward Super Users with financial incentives based on the utilization rate of physicians in their department or clinic.**

IS Support Team

> **Practice management analyst(s)**
> **Network administrator**
> **Server/Database administrator**
> **Client device support**
> **Application administrator**
> **Application support and/or Help-desk**

The Information Systems (IS) Support Team is the primary technical support for the Core Project Team during the implementation and rollout of the EHR, and also plays a prominent role in maintaining an effective, on-going operating environment for the EHR. In this role, the team members receive significant early support from the EHR vendor, especially in evaluating and implementing the necessary technical infrastructure, including the server environment, networking, and client device configuration.

The IS Support Team often drives the development of internal policies and procedures for the end-user support of the application, servers, network and associated devices. It's important to carefully consider who will fulfill this role because they must be people who are adept at interacting with clinicians and understanding their needs. For more details on individual roles within the IS Support Team, see Appendix One: Sample Resource Responsibilities and Qualifications.

Third-party vendors

Practice management system
Dictation system
Transcription system
Laboratory systems
Radiology systems
Pharmacies

Once the five project teams are in place, it's time to begin developing strong partnerships with the vendors who'll participate in the implementation. Although vendors don't report into your organization, it's your responsibility to ensure they meet their assigned deliverables. It is not uncommon for delayed deliverables from vendors to derail a project's momentum. Their involvement will be particularly critical to system configuration (base data /dictionary population), interface design, and integration testing. Three steps are essential to effectively managing third-party vendors. First, create a single point of contact within your organization—one individual who's responsible for communicating information to and from your vendors. Second, establish a clear escalation path for decisions and obstacles within your organization and the vendor organization. And third, clearly communicate expectations on deliverables and deadlines.

Step Two: Build the Right Roles for the Right People

For the EHR project to succeed, you need to help your team members be successful. Research and experience show that the best implementations are those that carefully design the project team's various roles and then fill them with people specifically chosen to succeed in each job. It's essential to avoid building jobs that require more skills or different experience than are possessed by the people you choose to fill them.

Once the appropriate people are chosen, it's important to dedicate the organization's resources to their success. Although many team members may be able to accomplish essential tasks on top of their current roles (super users, for example), in our experience the most effective approach, especially for the Core Project Team, is to create new jobs specific to the EHR implementation. Filling new jobs with your best people requires a serious commitment of resources on the part of your organization and a fully dedicated project team gives the work the focus and identity it needs to quickly and efficiently achieve the organization's strategic goals.

One of the most common missteps is to spend aggressively to purchase the best possible EHR but then resort to penny pinching when it comes time to implement and support it. There's nothing wrong with being frugal, of course. But heavy-handed efforts to conserve human resources may significantly delay the EHR's deployment and defeat its bottom-line returns, in the end costing you more than you save. The key, then, is to strike a balance between extravagance and stinginess.

The following suggestions will help you build and maintain strong project teams, no matter what level of resources you have at your fingertips:

- Some roles are flexible. In organizations of less than fifty physicians, several different combinations of team roles will support the goal of getting the work done in an economic fashion. A common area of consolidation for organizations of this size is in the IS Support Team, where a single person may serve as IS lead while also taking on several other support team roles, such as administering the network, server and database. Another common approach, especially in single-specialty practices, is to fill the role of Project Manager with someone who has extensive organizational experience within your clinics. The Project Manager could then serve as the Core Project Team's clinical and operational specialist, minimizing the number of other team members needed.
- Don't shortchange the Project Manager. The magnitude of coordination and change associated with implementing an EHR in organizations of all sizes is significant enough to warrant a full-time Project Manager for the duration. In fact, when the EHR is implemented using a phased approach, larger, multi-specialty organizations should consider allocating two Project Managers to accelerate the benefit of the EHR across the enterprise. In

this scenario, one Project Manager oversees the implementation of each new EHR module within designated showcase clinic(s), while a second PM works with leadership from the remaining clinics and specialties to deploy the module there. The two-pronged approach lets you implement new features quickly, which can greatly aid the all-important task of maximizing physician utilization of the system. Remember that a good Project Manager is essential to keeping your project on schedule and under budget while maximizing the new system's benefits to the organization. Without a dedicated Project Manager, the initiative risks limited success, if not outright failure. As Chapter Six outlined, it is also a good idea to try to find a Project Manager who has previous experience implementing an EHR.

- Don't under-resource technology. Another certain way to endanger the project is to fail to assign responsibility for designing, implementing and supporting an adequate technical foundation. It's not enough, however, to simply assign responsibility for the technology—you must also provide the chosen person with the appropriate training and resources they need to avoid becoming over-burdened. Few things will more adversely affect the willingness of your physicians to utilize the system than inadequate implementation and support of technology. The bottom line is, no matter how well the system's functionality is configured, if its performance negatively impacts clinical workflows, physicians will not use it.

- Training roles are flexible. The size of your organization and the breadth of your EHR will determine how many trainers you'll need to properly educate end-users. Only the very largest organizations need full-time trainers to support an implementation. Most organizations ask existing employees to take on the training role in addition to their current positions. You might look for trainers who possess clinical and business operations expertise, provided they have the appropriate teaching skills and time to fulfill the role. As subject matter experts, they can provide valuable early guidance in the design and configuration of the system workflows, and once all users are trained they can participate in post-live application support, add-on education sessions and/or administration of the application.

- Consider outsourcing end-user training. In larger organizations that already have a training department, temporarily outsourcing services can help supplement your existing resources, especially during periods of peak rollout to end-users. In smaller organizations, outsourcing training services can ensure that you engage the appropriate skilled staff to educate your end-users. When outsourcing education services, make sure that you plan appropriately for on-going training needs, such as application upgrades and new physicians and staff. (For details on outsourcing and other aspects of user training, see Chapter Nine—Making Users Comfortable and Productive From Day One).

- The IT department can't do everything. Another common mistake is to assume that IT workers should fill all project team roles because hardware and software are involved. The IT department in fact may fill a number of project team roles, but it's unlikely to have the resources to succeed in *all* the roles. Historically, those project teams that are made up of people from clinical and operational backgrounds have fared better than teams solely comprised of IT specialists.

- Executive Sponsors should provide strong governance. You get what you pay for when it comes to project teams. Strong teams properly nourished will deliver professional results. As an Executive Sponsor, it's your responsibility to assemble teams of the best people and to ensure they have the support and motivation they need to succeed. Unfortunately, the nurturing of project teams is commonly overlooked, with disastrous results in many cases. Executive Sponsors cannot simply assign work and then walk away. Even the most talented teams require executive leadership until they have grown into cohesive, high-performing machines. Even then, they will still require intermittent guidance and facilitation throughout the remainder of the project's lifecycle, in accordance with a clear project governance structure.

- It's not over 'til it's over. Even if you staff the initial install appropriately and have a wildly successful go-live event with your showcase clinics, that momentum will quickly stall if your overall EHR resource plan fails to sufficiently cover the on-going operational support needs of end users. A team built solely for the sprint without planning for the long run will inevitably fall apart due to the conflicting priorities of installation vs. on-going support. When you do not adequately staff for both of these priorities, members of your project team will by default be asked to provide support services to end-users while trying to implement new phases of the EHR. This will quickly compromise the success of both new and existing users and overextend your project teams' workload to such a degree that the schedule for further deployments becomes endangered. Worse, these problems risk triggering *reductions* in physician utilization of the system and elimination of the value returned to the organization from early physician use.

One glaring example of how *not* to plan for success comes from a recent implementation at a large, urban health care organization. The mistakes began right away with the assignment of the organization's help desk manager as EHR Project Manager. This immediately created three problems: a do-it-in-your-spare-time philosophy; lack of a dedicated Project Manager; and insufficient planning for end-user support. Because the Project Manager already supported many other systems on the help desk, she often found herself overwhelmed by day-to-day crises with little time left over for the EHR. The project eventually fell so far behind schedule that it became normal for several people to come in on weekends to build the system configuration. This approach not only created quality issues in the design of the configuration, but a ripple effect was felt after go-live when the help desk was so busy firefighting for new end-users of the EHR that they could not focus on the change-management needs of end-users (including on-going education and managerial coaching that would maximize physician utilization).

The organization eventually turned the project around by boosting the leadership's focus on project governance, and by hiring a full-time Project Manager. More time was allocated to design and validate system configuration, as well as to prepare and support end-users through the appropriate division of responsibility. After the implementation was complete, the Project Manager stayed on as a "change manager" to ensure that new workflows were well utilized and that the return to the organization was fully realized.

Step Three: Determine How Much (and Where) to Invest in the Project Team

Most organizations follow the same proven structure in designing the project team, but there's always variation in how resources are allocated to implement the structure. In our experience, the investment you make in the project team should be proportional to the outcomes you hope to achieve. For instance, if your organization hopes to realize a particularly large return over an accelerated timeframe, you may have to dedicate additional resources to the project, or supplement the existing skills within the organization.

To clarify the amount to invest in the project team, the Executive Sponsor should work with the finance department to quantify the expected outcomes of the EHR (for more on this subject, see Chapter Five, "Measuring ROI"). A clear understanding of the expected return on investment is important to justifying the resource costs required to succeed.

For guidance on base level staffing for each project team role, see Appendix One. The tables include comments specific to the size and complexity of the implementation.

Step Four: Finalize the Structure of Your Project Teams

Once you understand the framework for successful project teams and the work requirements for each role, you can begin to build a "straw man" resource structure for your organization's implementation. The plan should be validated to ensure that it supports the expected outcomes, sequencing and timeframe of your deployment strategy as well as your implementation and operational budgets. We also recommend that you review the plan with your EHR vendor to help identify gaps and provide potential improvements based on their experience. And don't forget to get the backing of your executive colleagues. You may need to rely on them for allocation of resources and/or presentation to your organization's board.

As you evaluate your straw man resource structure, take the time to identify those people in your organization that you would particularly like to leverage for the EHR implementation. Although care should be taken to avoid creating a vacuum elsewhere in the organization, some individuals may enhance the project's value by participating. Take the following considerations into account:

- What are their skills and are they unique?
- How available are they?
- Do they fit into a role within the proposed resource structure?
- Is there a logical modification to the resource structure that would allow you to benefit from this individual's special skills?
- How would the individual's current department be impacted by their reassignment?

In making your decision, be sure to consider the comparative value the individuals currently provide in other areas of the company and whether they can be effectively replaced. A clinic manger with prior deployment experience, for example, may be too valuable in their current role to commit to the project team on a full-time basis. But they might make a superb member of the EHR Steering Committee or effective part-time contributor to the local implementation at their clinic.

In order to attract the best and brightest to this exciting initiative, be sure to clearly communicate the importance and excitement surrounding the project, as well as potential career opportunities that could result from high performance. For example, your IS leader might seem like a perfect fit for some of the project's hands-on technical work and coordination. But he or she is likely to view such an assignment as a backward step on the career ladder, unless the project's importance is effectively conveyed.

Another consideration is the role of the Executive Sponsor in relating to the project team. It is recommended that certain responsibilities remain with the Executive Sponsor, including the primary (though not necessarily day-to-day) relationship with the EHR vendor, setting expected outcomes and deployment strategies, defining the project team's mission, and assessing the team's performance against that mission.

Step Five: Establish a System of Project Governance

Project Governance can be defined as the "set of structures, systems and processes around the project that assure the effective delivery of the project through to full utilization and benefits realization by the organization"(*World Project Management Week*, March 3, 2003). Key considerations for designing a project governance structure in a complex healthcare environment include the following:

- Involvement of the stakeholders most effected by implementation decisions
- Defined project success factors that serve as guiding principles for all go/no-go and other key decision points
- Identified key stakeholders for all decision points. Stakeholders should have authority (within the project governance structure) to recommend proposed decisions to the project team
- A balanced approach to project deliverables that considers project success criteria along with quality, cost and timeframe implications.
- Participation as the governance process changes. Participants move in and out of the model as the project progresses through various phases or stages.

EMR Project Governance Structure

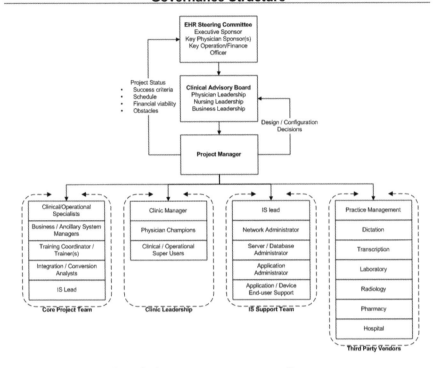

A typical governance structure diagram

Project Governance Structure

The governance structure pictured above has been adopted by many organizations but it may be customized to satisfy the nuances of your own organizational needs. Larger organizations, for instance, may want to plan for additional guidance from a clinical advisory board. Smaller organizations may skip the clinical advisory board and have a single Executive Sponsor replace the EHR Steering Committee. This model stresses the importance of defined roles, stakeholder involvement, clear escalation paths and swift issue resolution to continue forward momentum.

Below are the responsibilities and roles of each of the various project groups.

• The EHR Steering Committee is ultimately responsible for attainment of the overall project goals, objectives, success criteria, financial viability, as well as the removal of project obstacles throughout the organization (including within the governance structure). The Steering Committee is responsible for approving all design decisions, go/no-go decisions, the project plan, and the scope document.

- The Clinical Advisory Board, if utilized, is responsible for providing guidance and approval of system design and configuration decisions, as well as being an advocate of the system with their peers.

- The Project Manager(s) is accountable for coordinating all resources in the delivery of the project as defined in the Project Plan and Scope document (even though not all resources on work groups report to the PM), working within teams to remove obstacles when possible and escalating decisions up the governance structure when not possible.

- The Core Project Team is comprised of the Project Manager and individuals that represent the major areas of the project. They are the first team to evaluate change requests (scope, technical and/or functional) and push these requests through the other governing bodies if resolution cannot be achieved within the team.

- Work Group(s) are comprised of individuals assembled to provide input into the design, development and delivery of the implementation. If warranted, additional project teams can be created to focus on specific components of the implementation, such as system testing, conversion and interfaces, or education and adoption. A Core Project Team member would typically lead any additional workgroups created.

- Stakeholders should be identified within this structure for all key decision points: the Scope document, the project plan, and workflow design decisions. These stakeholders are responsible for validating recommendations made by the Core Project Team and providing recommendations when that group is not able to.

In addition to defining the roles of the team components, "escalation paths" for project deliverables should be clearly defined. An escalation path maps out the process for elevating an implementation decision or obstacle to a higher level in the project team structure when consensus can't be achieved at a lower level. Generally, the escalation path is from the project team and other teams to the Project Manager. If necessary, the Project Manager may escalate to the Core Project Team and then to the EHR Steering Committee or Clinical Advisory Board.

Scope Change Process

Project scope should be documented in a formal Project Scope Document. As described in the previous chapter, this deliverable identifies the goals, objectives, key deliverables, temporal scope, technical requirements, interface requirements and roles and responsibilities. The project plan should then be developed from the scope document. Both deliverables are reviewed and approved by the project Steering Committee. These documents become the guiding charter for the overall project.

Following the initial approval process, it may be necessary to expand or reduce the scope of the project. Changes to the scope document, project plan, design decisions, future policy/procedure documents, and other major project documentation deliverables should always go through a formal change-control process, described in Chapter Six. Change requests should be reviewed based upon their impact on project costs, timelines, available resources and their overall contribution to achieving the project success criteria. Most likely, these will be presented through the Project Manager and will need to be signed off or rejected by the Core Project Team and ultimately by the EHR Steering Committee/Executive Sponsor.

If the requested changes are approved, the scope document and project plan should be updated to reflect the changes and resources should be assigned appropriately to begin work on the change requests.

Step Six: Assemble Your Teams

Assembling the project teams is not as simple as it sounds. Gathering your team members while sticking to established organizational procedures is a fairly complex process that involves recruitment and transition policies, consideration of team dynamics, coordination with the HR department, and planning for a home base.

Recruitment and Transition

Job postings for the EHR implementation should clearly state expectations and appropriate qualifications. They should also stress the excitement and importance of the project to the organization. Postings should include clear guidance on whether appointments are permanent or temporary. If you have specific people in mind for certain roles, work through the appropriate channels to encourage those individuals to apply for the opportunity. Proactively pursue transition plans to speed the involvement of key people who move from other positions within the organization. If your organization needs to temporarily supplement your project team structure with outside resources, your EHR vendor may be able to help identify potential solutions.

Team Dynamics

Pay careful attention to the combination of individual personalities and skill sets that make up each team. A team with members from diverse backgrounds tends to perform better than a team of think-alike "yes-people," or one in which personality conflicts derail the team's capabilities. Ideally the team should be composed of:

- Task and/or detail-oriented individuals who provide solid technical or data-collection skills.
- Vision and goal-driven individuals willing to pitch in and work outside of assigned roles if needed.
- "People persons" who excel at communication, conflict-resolution, facilitation, and listening skills.
- Risk takers who question the status quo and encourage the team to take well-conceived risks to achieve improved results.

Human Resources

As teams are assembled and resources move to new positions or take on additional responsibility, work with your Human Resources department to evaluate potential compensation changes, implement new performance review criteria, and formalize training opportunities (e.g., training beyond the EHR solution, such as project management, wireless networking technologies, effective listening, and team facilitation skills).

Work Environment

Find a physical home base for the people who will be primarily responsible for implementing and supporting the deployment. Answer the questions: Does it make sense for people to be centralized? Is adequate space available with proper communications capabilities? What level of administrative support is available to the Core Project Team? At a minimum, the Core Project Team should have:

- Desk space/office supplies
- Client devices that meet minimum specifications for the EHR solution
- Network connectivity
- Phones/pagers
- Fax and printing capabilities
- Administrative support staff

Proactively tackling these important logistical issues will accelerate the assembly of the team and eliminate unnecessary misunderstandings and inefficiencies in the work environment.

Step Seven: Launch Your Teams

Once you have your teams in place, it's time to start their orientation. A welcome meeting or luncheon with executives or key stakeholders can be a good way to introduce team members and establish the significance and level of organizational support for the project.

Another effective tool is an internal project team orientation binder. This assists with getting new team members up to speed and as an ongoing reference for established team members. The orientation binder could include:

- A project organizational chart detailing the executive team, Core Project Team, IS Support Team and clinic leadership.
- A directory of contact information for ongoing communication.
- A list of each member's responsibilities to provide shared expectations and understanding.
- Clarification of who's available when, how to reach them, and what manner of reply to expect. Another useful place to house this information is a shared drive or Intranet page exclusively for the team's documentation.

Another recommended event to launch the EHR project team is a project team kick-off workshop. This meeting should be run by the Executive Sponsor and Physician Sponsor and is the right time and place to set high expectations for the project's schedule and overall quality. The primary objective is to educate the team about the project's objectives, measurable goals, standard deliverables, and suggested timeline. All team members should participate in team building and role-definition exercises, in which expectations can be clearly communicated with everyone present.

Once your internal planning and preparation is in place, you'll be more prepared to take advantage of the next steps with your EHR vendor, including a formal kick-off event with the vendor, education on the EHR solution and design sessions for system configuration. Once the project is underway, the Executive Sponsor and Project Manager should meet periodically with each project team member to make sure they're comfortable in their role, assess any training needs, and ensure that they're scheduled with the appropriate workload moving forward.

VITALS

Soon after forming the project team, set expectations through an internal project team kick-off workshop. This session will build momentum for team members by clarifying goals and expectations.

Step Eight: Develop your Teams

New teams don't become high-performance engines the day after they're assembled. It takes time for teams to form cohesive units. The process can be sped up by assigning them, early on, reasonably easy "mini-deliverables" that strengthen the team's muscles before they're called on to do the heavy lifting of mission-critical deliverables such as project design and planning documents.

In developing your teams, it's helpful to understand the fundamentals of team dynamics. The most widely accepted model of group dynamics recognizes four developmental stages: "forming, storming, norming, and performing" (this theory was developed in the 1960s by Bruce W. Tuckman, a professor of educational psychology at Ohio State University). When a team is first assembled, according to Tuckman's model, participants are excited by the freshness of the endeavor, and tend to be polite and pleasant with one another. This is the early "forming" stage, a sort of team honeymoon. Next, the team moves into an end-of-the-honeymoon "storming" phase in which individuals begin testing one another and asserting their own ideas and values. Teams that survive the storming phase begin to feel more comfortable with each other, more normal. Finally, the team reaches the "performing" stage of mutual trust, with a shared agreement that the team's mission is more important than its individual members.

By assembling your Core Project Team and Steering Committee early, ideally during the sales process, you buy them time to work through the four stages of team development. During the project's early stages, the Executive

Sponsor must provide leadership and direction to give the team a proper sense of its mission and boundaries. The Executive Sponsor should also look for ways to test the team before it's first major project deliverables are due. The Executive Sponsor could, for instance, require the core team to draft a project charter outlining the major goals, success criteria, metrics, and plan for pre-live and post-live ROI measurements. The team could then present the document to the Executive Sponsor and the Steering Committee. A second test might be to ask the team to author and present a project management/governance plan. By the time the team has passed these early tests, they'll be ready to move on to the critical early implementation phases.

Step Nine: Monitor, Evaluate and Facilitate Progress

Once teams have assembled, received clear direction and begun to establish healthy team dynamics, the role of the Executive Sponsor transitions from establishing boundaries and expectations to monitoring and facilitating team progress. By maintaining active communications with each of the project's components (Core Project Team, Steering Committee, etc.) and with vendors, the Executive Sponsor can facilitate resolution of any significant problems that might otherwise threaten the progress or credibility of the project.

One way for the Executive Sponsor to maintain healthy communications with the entire team structure is to conduct monthly executive status reviews. The reviews can be co-sponsored by your internal Project Manager and the vendor's Project Manager. Active participation in the reviews will help the Executive Sponsor to measure progress and identify and remove obstacles. These interactions also will uncover early evidence of team success (meeting project deadlines, major project milestones, etc.), which should be widely publicized to build confidence and excitement within the organization.

Let's return again to the benefit of tying financial metrics to physician utilization and other outcomes, and how to leverage them to evaluate and facilitate progress. To the extent that metrics can be devised for expected value returned to the organization, the numbers will give the project teams clear guidelines for prioritizing their efforts. Make sure the metrics are as specific as possible. For example, an objective that quantifies workflow improvements will help focus the attention of the physician community as well as the teams who are responsible for implementing system features that help realize that return. In this example, the organization could even decide to implement further incentives for the workflow objective by giving physicians a deadline for either utilizing the system or paying their own transcription costs.

Step Ten: Maintain a Motivational Environment

The timeframe for completion of your deployment enterprise-wide will vary based on the size and complexity of your organization and the functionality being implemented. Whether it takes six months or eighteen months, it's important to keep the people on your project teams motivated and energized.

To this end, we recommend that performance plans be implemented as appropriate, and that compensation plans be developed for people who are expected to make significant contributions to the effort. Depending on the individual, there are several potential metrics to leverage in compensation plans, which can be either reward-based or penalty-based incentives. These include:

- Successfully meeting project milestone dates and/or producing quality deliverables (such as new process design documents, training curriculum, test plans, etc).
- Getting a set percentage of physicians to utilize the system by a given date.
- Measured value returned to the organization through project execution.

Many resources may have left other career paths to work on the EHR project. By providing them ongoing training and personal development opportunities, the organization demonstrates its investment in them. Ultimately, the investment in such perks will be returned to the organization through hard work.

Even with the ingredients in place for a highly motivational working environment, however, attrition will still occur. To keep departing team members from taking critical knowledge with them, promote the development of "organizational memory" as part of your culture. By requiring documentation of tools used, lessons learned and policies and procedures created, you assure that the team's knowledge pool won't have to be rebuilt upon every departure.

The Recap

- Understand the components of successful EHR project teams. Each component of the EHR project team structure fulfills a vital role in the planning, decision-making and advocacy of the project.
- Learn from the experience of others. Solicit input from your EHR vendor through a deployment strategy assessment, peer organizations and the increasing volume of case studies published on the Internet.

- Determine the number of resources needed for your organization. This planning is critical to the budgeting process, and to building awareness throughout the organization and emphasizing the importance of the initiative by highlighting the effort required across the organization.

- Finalize your organization's project team structure. Combine the roles, responsibilities and skills associated with the major components of a successful project team structure with the resource estimates for your organization to formulate a staffing plan. This plan will provide a focused structure for your recruiting efforts for this vital initiative.

- Formalize and document your system of project governance. It is important that each role within your project team structure understand from the beginning how decisions will be made, their role in the decision-making process, as well as when and how decisions will be escalated.

- Assemble your teams. Closely evaluate candidates for their ability to fulfill the responsibilities of the roles in your staffing plan, taking into consideration team dynamics, the impact on other areas of the organization and human resources factors.

- Launch your team! Although some resources in your EHR project team structure may have had prior involvement in preparing to launch the initiative, it is important to launch the initiative with all participants to create a common awareness of the objectives, its importance to the organization and excitement to springboard the project.

- Develop your core project team into a cohesive, high-performing unit. This process rarely occurs spontaneously and requires focused time and attention from the executive and physician sponsors early in the project.

- Monitor, evaluate and facilitate progress. The executive and physician sponsors are responsible for ensuring that acceptable progress is being made against the organizations objectives and for taking the appropriate actions to balance organizational acceptance with the project budget and timeline.

- Maintain a motivating environment. Executive and physician sponsors need to continually build a motivating environment by highlighting the goal, and providing continual feedback and career growth opportunities for core project team members who may have left another role in the organization to wok on the EHR initiative.

If You Have Time

"Developmental Sequence in Small Groups," by B.W. Tuckman. Psychological Bulletin, vol. 63, 1965, pp. 384–399.

CHAPTER EIGHT

Going Paperless: Key Design Considerations

In This Chapter
- Build paperless workflows
- Enable reduced chart pulls
- Design to reduce physician dictation
- Convert data and load content
- Integrate with other systems

Modern healthcare occasionally seems to be an odd blend of state-of-the-art technology and century's-old procedures. Just consider. A patient who undergoes an MRI—one of the world's most advanced diagnostic tests—often has the results noted by hand in a paper chart that must be photocopied to be shared. One explanation for this disjunction is that the transition to a paperless medical record is a complex undertaking that requires planning far in advance of implementation.

Much of that planning surrounds the assessment of current work processes, or workflows, to determine whether they are transferable to an EHR. The answer is not always cut and dried. For instance, some paper workflows can't be performed electronically and some electronic processes work better on paper. Divining the difference requires taking a situation-by-situation approach to analyzing your organization's workflows before designing them into an EHR. The same is true of virtually every other aspect of EHR design. Simplistic answers lead to simplistic functionality—and eventually many of reluctant users.

In this chapter we'll present some of the most important design factors to take into account before implementing an EHR.

Special Considerations for Paperless Workflows

Just as workflows vary from one organization to the next, an EHR's functionality can be quite different, too. One organization's physician dictations may be included in the EHR; another's may not. One may have lab results built into the system; another may still rely on paper scripts. While the EHR's great strength is its flexibility, the truly complete electronic health record is *completely* paperless—all clinical data is populated in the EHR and the paper chart is archived. However, not every organization will be able to adopt a full EHR.

How do you determine whether your organization is ready to go paperless? Ask yourself whether your users would be able to adjust to viewing clinical data online vs. reading a piece of paper. If you're confidant the answer is yes, then your organization is already well on its way to a paperless workflow.

Still, making the decision to pursue a full EHR isn't the same as preparing the ground for it to happen. For an organization to become truly paperless, several important design decisions must first be made. We'll run through them one at a time.

Identify Locations Where the Electronic Chart Will Be Accessed

Determine the need for physical access to the electronic chart. If the paper chart is going to be removed, it's vital that the electronic chart is easily accessed. One common way to accomplish this is to place networked desktop computers with access to the HER in every exam room and area pod. If wireless networking is available, then the clinical staff can access the electronic chart in virtually any area of the facility using Tablet PCs or PDAs.

Physicians often take a paper chart with them when they visit patients in the hospital. Once the paper chart is gone, your organization must enable physicians to access the electronic record offsite. Some organizations accomplish this by providing offline access through mobile devices such as a PDA, which store the record between regular updates, or by designating a secure workstation at the hospital that providers can use to access the EHR. We recommended that you work with your EHR vendor to identify features and configuration options to accommodate these workflows through stationary or mobile devices in the hospital. (For more on this topic, see Chapter Eleven).

Review All Paper Processes for Efficacy Before Conversion

In general, the workflows supported by paper processes are simplistic—a paper form is transmitted and an action is performed. To achieve a paperless workflow, each of these paper processes should be weighed for inclusion in the EHR. The sorting of mail is a good example. In a paper system, a nurse or office manager reviews incoming mail and discards unneeded information without the physicians' review. When an EHR is deployed, the organization may choose to have the nurse or office manager continue to review the mail before scanning or simply scan all mail into the system. The decision impacts whether all data is memorialized to portions of the patient chart, and whether human interaction is still needed to pre-filter the documents. It's a good opportunity to review existing processes and redesign future ones.

An example of an existing paper process on the clinical side is the medication renewal process. Today, a medical renewal request may include the following steps:

- The patient's request is received via phone or fax.
- The message is transmitted to the appropriate clinician via paper or e-message.
- The chart is pulled to review existing medications.
- Approval of the refill is granted.
- The refill request is transmitted to the pharmacy (usually by fax).
- The refill approval is documented in the patient's chart.
- The patient's chart is sent back to the medical records department.

When this process is converted to an EHR, the organization must determine the procedures to be used for capturing and routing the message, accessing the chart reviewing existing medications, calling in the refill and documenting the approval. The decision impacts whether all data is captured to portions of the paper chart and whether human interaction is still needed to maintain this information.

Before converting an existing paper process, it's advisable to examine the efficacy of the workflow, to fix bad processes and redesign others. In other words, ask yourself what steps should be taken to ensure that a particular paper workflow is appropriately translated into an electronic workflow. Some paper workflows can't be performed electronically and some electronic processes just work better on paper.

For example, a physician might be accustomed to initialing lab results and placing them in an outbox for routing by a clerk. When this workflow is converted into the EHR, the physician is still responsible for viewing and initialing the lab result, and determining routing. However the process now requires the use of a keyboard and mouse; so it's likely to be even more time consuming than the old paper process.

Many methodologies offer guidance on the workflow analysis process. Guidelines specified in "The Power of Six Sigma," by Subir Chowdhury, have been used successfully by many organizations to analyze the efficacy of their existing workflows. The title comes from the mathematical symbol for standard deviation, "sigma," which is a measure of variation. According to the Six Sigma guidelines, a process is efficient when the number of defective results it produces is small enough to fit within six standard deviations of the mean performance and an acceptable specification limit).

The Six Sigma process begins with the following steps:

- Define the problem. Measure current performance by collecting data and creating metrics.
- Analyze to identify root causes.
- Improve by eliminating root causes.
- Control by making permanent changes and reviewing.

The Six Sigma process suggests that before you can ensure that a paper workflow is appropriate for conversion into an electronic workflow, you must first understand, document, and measure your current processes.

Acknowledge That You May Use More Paper After Implementation

Before going "paperless" with an EHR, consider some policy decisions that could prevent paper use from actually increasing—at least temporarily—with the new system. Dr. Richard M. Podhajny noted this strange phenomenon in an article in Paper, Film & Foil Converter, a monthly Internet printing magazine. "It wasn't too long ago that the coming of the electronic age was predicted to have dire effects on the use of paper," Podhanjny wrote. "In fact, the opposite has occurred. The predictions for the demise of paper demand failed to appreciate the fact that the average person wants a 'hard copy.'"

We all know the truth of this observation. The low cost of electronic information retrieval—and a general failure to consider the costs of printing—makes it easier for employees to use more paper than in the past. The EHR should reduce paper filing in the long term, but expect to see an increase in paper use immediately following implementation as employees print out paper reference manuals and other reference information. Paper consumption can be expected to drop over time as users become more comfortable retrieving and storing information electronically.

Some organizations have implemented policies and procedures that discourage employees from printing unnecessarily, including:

Implement faxing alternatives: In a paper system, incoming faxes are scanned and indexed into the patient chart. In implementing its EHR's scan functionality, Orthopedic Associates USA designed the system to save incoming faxes to a server in digital form. This step eliminated the need for printing all incoming faxes before scanning, saving the organization $6,000 on paper and ink in the first six months alone.

Use a workflow engine (tasking): If your organization's EHR enables the electronic communication of tasks, consider mapping out existing workflows so they can be incorporated into the system. Incorporating everyday workflows in an electronic setting generally reduces the need to print certain tasks or documents because they are captured electronically.

Establish Organization-Wide Printing Guidelines

Organizations may choose to strongly encourage their employees to use terminals vs. printing by assigning printing responsibility to different people. This approach has proven most successful when printing is shifted from the clerical staff to the doctor's nurse. For example, it's common for a physician who refuses to use the EHR to require the medical records department to continue printing the last office note. If the responsibility for printing the note were shifted to the physician's nurse, however, the nurse would be forced to stop clinical care to pull and print the chart. In the interest of protecting patient care, the printing requests would soon cease.

Stop Distributing the Paper Chart Once All Information Has Been Captured by the EHR

Some organizations may choose to reinforce the switch to an EHR by creating policies that prohibit printing of the chart. To increase their effectiveness, such policies should be reviewed with employees, allowing time for questions or voicing of concern.

Before you implement strict paper-control policies, be sure to consider your organization's culture and size. At least one organization that implemented a nurse-only printing policy had to abandon it after employees voiced frustration with their lack of control over this simple task. Other organizations were able to successfully implement a similar policy, despite initial employee frustration, by convincing staff that the new policy supported important organizational goals.

Identify Changing Roles Used to Capture Clinical Data

Another design factor that should be decided before going paperless concerns how data is entered into the EHR. With the onset of more direct data entry into a patient's chart, organizations may find that the employees who historically captured information in the patient's paper chart no longer are required to do so in the EHR. On the other hand, resources may be assigned responsibility for entering data electronically that they were not responsible for in the paper chart.

For example, physicians may be accustomed to dictating a patient's visit, receiving a hard copy of the transcribed text, reviewing the transcription for accuracy and sending it back to the transcriptionist for corrections. With an EHR, physicians may receive the transcribed text electronically and be responsible for making the corrections themselves within the EHR. The increase in efficiency of the workflow translates into more direct involvement in editing by the physician, and is a factor organizations must consider when identifying workflows.

Acknowledge That Required Skill Levels May Increase as the Number of Resources Decreases

In preparing to go paperless with an EHR, you should understand how the change will impact your most important resource—the people who'll use it. Because an EHR is so much more efficient than paper records, it can sharply reduce the number of people needed for filing and pulling paper charts. Central Utah Clinic (CUM) experienced this phenomenon in 2003, when several members of the medical records department were laid off or moved to other jobs following an EHR implementation.

In switching to an EHR, the skill level required of medical records' personnel might actually increase. That's because the new process of entering paper-based information into the EHR generally requires two steps: physically scanning the document and then indexing it to the appropriate patient or folder. While a college intern or other temporary resource can scan the documents, it takes someone with clinical experience to do the indexing properly and to review questionable documents to see whether they were misfiled. (On a related note, if you purchase an EHR for its scanning capability, be sure that it allows you to change or move documents that are mistakenly scanned into the wrong patient's chart or the wrong folder).

Organize Document Categories for Efficient, Easy Viewing

The final design factor to consider before you go paperless is how to increase the efficiency of viewing documents in the EHR. A typical EHR offers a variety of ways that data may be filtered and viewed by users. These include sorting documents chronologically, sorting documents according to user defaults based on who is logged into the system, and allowing physicians from different specialties to view only those documents generated within their department (e.g., cardiology vs. internal medicine). (For more information on the viewing functionality of an EHR, see Chapter Two, "The EHR Mental Model").

There are steps you can take to design the most efficient views possible. Consider taking the following steps ahead of implementation:

- Minimize the number of documents a user needs to access before finding the desired information. If the descriptions of the documents are too vague or include too many different types of data, the user will end up scrolling through many different documents before finding the correct one. Ensure that the document names are descriptive enough to tell the user what's inside.

- Identify the appropriate number of document types to use in storing and retrieving documents within the viewer. Deciding whether your document names should be more complex or less complex depends on the type of EHR you purchase. Many top-of-the-line EHR's can filter and search documents by specialty, document type or other criteria. If your EHR has this capability, you don't need to worry about using complex naming conventions to make it easy for users to identify the proper document—the EHR will search the entire contents of the document for the proper information, not just the document name. In this case, you should consider simplifying the document naming conventions to make searches more efficient. If your EHR does not have the ability to filter and search by specific criteria, then you should ensure that the document type names are sufficiently descriptive to help the end-user find the right document. For example, within the paper chart, a multi-specialty organization may use "office notes" as a document type. When building document types for viewing, consider adding specificity to the document type name by including the provider's medical specialty so that a cardiologist knows to look for the "cardiology office note" vs. the "orthopedic office note." Otherwise, he or she would need to search for all such documents in order to find the notes specific to cardiology. .

- Devote time and resources to proper document labeling during the indexing process. As discussed above, scanning documents into an EHR is usually a two-step process: scanning the document and then indexing it to the appropriate patient or folder. During the indexing process it's wise to encourage the administrative staff to devote as much time as necessary to creating highly specific document type names. In the short-term, it may seem like a waste of time, but in the long-term the more descriptive document type names will save end-users—and the organization—far more time than it cost to create them.

Strategies for Reducing Paper Chart Pulls

When implementing an EHR, the ideal situation would be to have every page of every patient's chart scanned into the new system. That way, there would no longer be any need for storing, filing and pulling the old paper chart—everything would be electronic. However practical considerations, such as cost, make this situation highly unlikely. In the absence of a totally digital chart, several questions must be answered before the EHR comes online:

- Should you scan all historical information into the EHR? The charts of long-term patients may consist of multiple folders. How much of that history should be considered important enough to scan into the EHR? The answer is important because an incomplete EHR chart leads to more requests to pull the paper chart for review, which contributes to higher operational costs.

- Should existing electronic data processes be converted into the EHR? If your organization captures data electronically from a transcription or lab company, you should consider converting the process into the EHR.

- How much of the chart should you scan and index? The decision to scan a patient's chart requires an organization to decide whether the entire chart should be scanned, or only designated portions. Once it's scanned, you must then determine how much of the scanned chart should be indexed and how much filed directly into a folder.

The majority of organizations scan only those portions of the active chart that they feel are most important. Determining how much to scan often becomes a question of balancing the financial benefits of going paperless with the clinical benefits of maintaining the entire paper chart for physician review. This quandary can spark a tug-of-war between the physicians and the administration, which may argue that physicians rarely use the historical chart, so why keep it? The clear answer—and a best practice—is that organizations should simply do what's right and scan the entire chart, but only index a portion of the chart.

Strategies for Reducing, Streamlining and Eliminating Physician Dictation/Transcription

As health care costs continue to rise, medical transcription is an easy target for cost cutting. Increasing demands on physicians' time coupled with increased documentation requirements have led healthcare facilities to spend an estimated 20 billion dollars annually on medical transcription services, according to the American Association for Medical Transcription. In an attempt to reduce this expense, healthcare administrators have focused on solutions that attempt to boost transcriptionist efficiency, but these efforts have met with limited success.

An alternative to focusing on transcription-based efficiencies is to leverage technology to seamlessly document clinical encounters. Leading practices have found that a properly planned, modular implementation of an EHR is a highly effective change-management strategy that enables healthcare organizations to significantly reduce or eliminate transcription. Short of an EHR, several products and strategies exist that will either improve the responsiveness and efficiency of dictation/transcription; combine dictation with other methods to reduce transcription or eliminate dictation/transcription all together. These include:

Mobile Digital Dictation

Wireless digital dictation devices, such as handheld PDAs and Tablet PCs, give physicians access to a patient list, and can add efficiencies and quality to traditional dictation and transcription processes. Physicians can dictate clinical notes into the convenient devices, saving 20 to 30 seconds per patient encounter. Most mobile solutions also automatically attach demographics and other patient data to the recording, reducing the number of lines that need to be transcribed and accelerating turnaround time. Mobile devices can further reduce dictation by advising the physician on the degree of documentation required for each visit. And when they are integrated into an EHR, these advanced mobile solutions provide a complete solution—immediate access to real-time patient information, the status of the current encounter, and access to the completed note.

Structured Note Templates

Combining dictation with structured note templates can significantly reduce the volume of dictation. Physicians increasingly use electronic templates loaded with boilerplate information for standard sections of the clinical note—information they would otherwise have to cite or obtain from the patient record. Templates allow physicians to dictate only the most important sections of the note. Leading EHRs come pre-loaded with templates utilizing medical terminology from coding sources like MEDCIN(r). This allows the EHR to also provide clinical decision support during the patient encounter. Taken together, templates and dictation can reduce transcription to just a few sentences per encounter, saving time for the physician and transcription charges for the practice. Additionally bringing templates into a mobile environment achieves the dual benefits of wireless digital dictation with structured documentation.

Speech Recognition

In recent years, as the quality of speech recognition software has improved, front-end speech recognition has thrived in specific clinical specialties such as radiology. Front-end speech recognition, which shows up on a computer screen at the time of dictation and can be corrected by the physician, is increasingly being used to augment structured notes in an EHR. Because real-time documentation eliminates transcription costs, more practices are finding ways to encourage physicians to incorporate speech recognition technology.

In contrast to front-end speech recognition, the back-end version of the technology lets physicians dictate and run, just like the old phone-based systems. Transcriptionists correct the recognition, achieving an average 25 to 30 percent gain in efficiency over standard transcription. Because back-end speech recognition requires no change in physician behavior, it tends to be more popular than the front-end technology. While both solutions require a significant investment along with a substantial workflow change for transcriptionists, many large transcription services have proven willing to absorb the costs in exchange for added efficiencies.

Workflow Integration

The ultimate solution for documenting clinical encounters relies on workflow integration and documentation capture as part of a more complete EHR. Workflow integration automatically collects patient data entered into either a practice management system or an EHR and then uses the data to populate the clinical note during the patient care process. By leveraging existing data and allowing the documentation to be built during the patient encounter across physicians, clinicians, and nursing staff, the documentation process is streamlined and constructed in a manner that mirrors the delivery of healthcare.

Many leading practices are finding ways to seamlessly document clinical encounters while encouraging physician adoption of these electronic solutions by initially requiring few behavioral changes of them. Managing documents through mobile, wireless dictation and anytime-anywhere access to the completed note moves organizations closer to implementing a full EHR. Once physicians begin to appreciate the efficiencies from this initial step, they tend to migrate towards a structured note approach, further reducing transcription expense. A number of physician practices have already implemented this model of clinical notation with impressive results.

A Case in Point

Central Utah Clinic leveraged an EHR to help control their transcription costs and to bring additional efficiencies to their organization. CUC initially enabled their physicians to use a PDA to dictate anywhere and anytime. This gave the practice's physicians an easy way to dictate and better access to patient information.

CUC then introduced the note functionality of their EHR, enabling physicians to document in the exam room at the point of care and eliminating transcription costs for many. CUC's physicians also commonly augment the template process with front-end speech recognition that inserts text directly into subjective sections of the note. Thanks to templates and speech recognition, physicians were able to leave work earlier with more detailed documentation, and to document higher coding levels—all while eliminating dictation costs.

As reported in the Winter 2004 issue of the *Journal of Healthcare Information Management*, the change has produced significant savings for CUC. The practice estimates it will save $660,000 on transcription costs in 2004, and nearly $5 million over five years. The EHR has also allowed CUC to reduce chart pulls by 40 percent and to improve coding levels thanks to improved documentation practices. The practice is currently building a completely paperless new facility that lacks a chart room. Following these preliminary results, CUC has added additional modules for orders, accessing lab results, prescribing and even capturing charges.

As you can see, the transcription-documentation challenge today goes well beyond the application of transcription management tools that merely automate an inefficient dictation and transcription process. Such solutions only partially address the costs of clinical documentation. But by focusing on physician workflows and how clinical documentation can be aligned with an EHR, healthcare organizations can significantly improve the documentation of clinical encounters, enhancing accuracy and patient safety, and achieving real reductions in the cost of transcription.

Strategies for Loading Content into the EHR

In Chapter Three, we discussed the design and input of EHR clinical content from the physician's perspective (specifically, pick lists and patient data). Here we will discuss some of the technical aspects of converting *existing* digital information into the EHR. To begin, consider the following questions: Do you currently capture elements of a patient record electronically? If you do, then do you first review the integrity of the source data to determine if it makes sense to convert it into electronic form? Is your organization interested in reducing chart pulls when the EHR goes live?

If you answered yes to any of these questions, then the electronic components of your source system may be eligible for conversion into the EHR. Conversion automates the transfer of data from the old system into the EHR, as opposed to physically typing the data into the new system. Converting data from an existing information system to the EHR is usually far more efficient than manually entering it, but be aware that it may impact the usability of the new system.

To determine if pursuing a data-conversion strategy is worthwhile, consider doing the following:

- **Perform a cost/benefit analysis.** If source data exists in electronic format, your organization must determine the cost effectiveness of conversion versus manually entering it into the EHR. A simple analysis would estimate the time it takes to manually enter the data and then prices the time accordingly, taking into consideration possible overtime pay and reductions in revenue due to employees neglecting their current jobs to complete the data entry.

- **Determine how much and what type of data to convert.** Your clinical team can determine the type of data to be converted and decide how far back in time to go in retrieving it. Information on patient medications, for instance, may be needed for the previous year, while six months' worth of lab results may be enough. The guideline is to choose data that helps your organization make clinical decisions that are medically necessary for continuity of care.

- **Assess the integrity of the source data.** Prior to pursuing a data conversion strategy, consider reviewing the source data to ensure that it's accurate and up-to-date. Many organizations pursue a clean-up effort to reduce duplicate records and remove inactive entries prior to data conversion.

Integrating with External Systems

Connecting your EHR to external information systems such as a practice management system or laboratory often makes it easier to maintain a complete and current patient chart. Once integrated, the external systems can automatically populate the chart with current data that would otherwise have to be manually entered. Typical system integrations include:

- **ADT (Admissions, Discharges and Transfers) information.** Provided by hospitals via a live feed, ADT information can be used to auto-populate the patient list and provide up-to-date information on patient status.

- **Practice Management Systems (PMS).** The PMS provides registration, scheduling and billing information critical for adding or updating demographic, insurance, and appointment information for the patient.

- **Laboratory and radiology data.** Two-way integration allows you to either send outbound radiology and lab orders via the EHR, or receive inbound results that are automatically entered in the patient chart.

- **Transcription suppliers.** Integration can route digital voice files from the EHR's dictation module directly to the transcription service.

- **PACS systems.** Organizations may choose to integrate with a Picture Archiving and Communication System (PACS) to populate imaging results into the EHR. Integration lets providers view the image side by side with the clinical note.

- **Medical devices.** Many devices can integrate with an EHR. For example, a Welch Allyn device that is used to test blood pressure, temperature, oxygen-saturation and heart rate can electronically share the information with the EHR (or any computer) through a standard interface. This information instantly appears in the appropriate patient's record for reference by end-users.

- **Patient eHealth systems.** Patient eHealth systems let patients request appointments or prescription renewals, and update registration information over the Internet via secure messaging. Integration captures patient requests (e.g., for medication renewals) and documents the action in the EHR without additional data entry.

The benefits of integrating the EHR with external information systems are clear, but the strategy can also be expensive. Before deciding whether integration with a particular external system makes sense for your organization, run through the following list of questions:

- Is the external source compatible with the EHR?
- Does the external system help provide ease of access to patient data?
- Does the external system provide data that is indispensable to performing patient care?

- What are the costs and financial benefits of building an interface with the external system?

- Are there alternative ways to capture the information, such as manual entry of lab results?

The answers to these questions should make it easy for you to decide on a case-by-case basis whether integration makes sense.

The Recap

- Going paperless requires careful planning. Begin by determining where the new electronic chart will be physically accessed in your facility.

- Assess individual paper-based workflows carefully to see whether they merit inclusion in the EHR as electronic workflows. Six Sigma principles will help to understand, document and measure your current processes. This is a good opportunity to examine the efficacy of each workflow, to fix bad processes and design new, improved processes.

- Design the EHR to view documents more efficiently by: minimizing the number of documents a user must access before finding the desired information; identifying the appropriate number of document types to use in storing and retrieving documents within the viewer; label the documents appropriately during the indexing process

- Reduce the need for paper chart pulls by scanning the entire medical chart into the EHR rather than only certain portions of it.

- Make use of technologies and strategies that will either improve the responsiveness and efficiency of dictation/transcription, combine dictation with other methods to reduce transcription, or eliminate dictation/transcription. These include mobile digital dictation, structured note templates, speech recognition and workflow integration.

- Before deciding whether existing digital data should be converted into the EHR you should determine the cost effectiveness of conversion versus manually entering the data into the new system. Be sure to examine the source data for accuracy.

- Integrating the EHR with external systems (laboratory systems, PACS, etc.) offers advanced functionality but may be expensive. Conduct a separate cost-benefit analysis of each integration before proceeding; you may find that alternative data-capture methods such as data entry are more cost-effective.

If You Have Time

- Strategies and Technologies for Healthcare Information: Theory Into Practice. Marion J. Ball, Judith V. Douglas, Douglas E. Garets, and David E. Garets. Springer-Verlag (1999).

CHAPTER NINE

Making Users Comfortable and Productive from Day One

It's probably safe to assume by now that you have decided to purchase the EHR, worked through the budgets and put the project plan in place. All the required interfaces have been identified, resources have been allocated, and the groundwork seems to be set for a trouble-free implementation.

However, while everything may be in place from the standpoint of technical, functional and logistical requirements, we have not yet discussed the most important component of any major implementation or change—the users. If your organization wants to achieve all the benefits of the new EHR, your people have to use it.

If that sounds obvious, it's not. The most common reason for an EHR implementation to falter is not technical; it's that people who are accustomed to the old way of doing things never really accept the new. Which is why we keep returning to a key principle of this book, IDDUINEM (If Doctors Don't Use It, Nothing Else Matters).

In this chapter we'll give you the tools you need to ensure that your organization's users accept, even *embrace*, the changes that the new EHR will introduce. Properly preparing for change is the vital first step on the path towards making your users comfortable and productive. We begin with a plan of attack for the first hurdle on that path—fear of change.

Preparing for Change

Preparing for change would seem to be an obvious component of any major project but, oddly, organizations of all kinds commonly overlook this critical step. The assumption seems to be that simply implementing a system and demanding that it be used will result in effective utilization. Unfortunately, demands and threats are rarely effective at getting users to incorporate new technology into their daily workflows. One big reason: Change is scary. No matter how motivated new users are to improve patient safety, save time and money, and support all the other beneficial aspects of an EHR, their good intentions can whither in the face of troubling unanswered questions. What if I look stupid? What if I don't *get* it? What if I lose data? Will this make my job more difficult? Will I be as effective as I am now? Will it make my job less secure? Or, I signed on to help people—why do I have to learn about computers?

Whether spoken or unspoken, these are natural fears that must be addressed if your organization is to be properly prepared for the coming change. It won't do any good to pretend the fears aren't real, or to hastily reason them away. As with all fears, the prerequisite for overcoming them is to first acknowledge their existence and their validity. After all, there's good reason to be afraid of change—it's disruptive, unruly and occasionally traumatic. Thankfully, there are strategies that can help manage the troubling nature of change and soothe the fears that come with it.

To nip user fear in the bud, we recommend three key strategies:

• Establish Executive Sponsorship

• Conduct a Cultural/Educational Assessment

• Develop the Communication Plan

Establish Executive Sponsorship

The importance of the Executive Sponsor has been highlighted in previous chapters, so we will not cover it in depth here. But one other critical component of the Executive Sponsor's role deserves to be mentioned here. Few people care to invest the time and energy necessary to use a new technology unless they first understand why it's important. For that reason, user training should include not only *how* to use the newly implemented EHR but *why*. In other words, what led the executive team to invest the organization's time, money and resources into implementing an EHR? Experience has shown that the most effective way to deliver this message to front-line workers is through the Executive Sponsor. Doing so immediately highlights the importance of user acceptance of the EHR, and deflates the naysayers and change-resistors who might otherwise cast doubt on the organization's commitment to the new system.

Assess the Organization's Culture and Users' Educational Needs

A cultural and educational assessment lets you know how much work you have to do to prepare your organization for the coming changes. The cultural component of the assessment determines whether your organization is change-ready or change-resistant. If it's change-ready—meaning that the workforce is flexible, adaptable, and excited by new prospects and the idea of change—then you're not only in good shape for your implementation, you are also definitely in the minority. If the opposite is true, and your organization thwarts or actively resists change, then you've got your work cut out for you and again you are in the minority.

The truth is that most people are somewhere in the middle—they understand the need for change and are willing to make the necessary adjustments but they're still a little bit afraid of the results. In the language of technology adoption, this group is known as the "early and late majority" (see "Understanding the Adoption Curve"). Because they comprise by definition the largest number of users, in this chapter we'll focus primarily on making this group comfortable with the coming change.

The educational component of the cultural/educational assessment is designed to gain an understanding of the "skill readiness" of your organization for this EHR implementation. For example, are basic computer skills are in place? For many of us, double-clicking with a mouse is second nature but you shouldn't assume that all of your nursing staff is computer literate. Here we're talking about simple familiarity: Do they know how to use a mouse, toggle between fields, move between documents and programs, etc.? Before you can introduce specific EHR functionality, you should ensure that your staff knows the difference between a laptop and a PDA, a Web browser and Solitaire, storm windows and Microsoft Windows. Assuming the basic computer skills are present when they are not will not only further frighten your users, it may severely delay project milestones and utilization progress.

The educational assessment also will help identify the various personnel roles that need to be educated on the EHR and the related workflow processes. Understanding how your users will employ the EHR within their daily workflow is critical to determining the training content and its delivery.

Below is an example of a typical cultural/educational assessment. Candid consideration of each of the components and questions within this assessment will help you identify and understand the barriers to change as well as the tools you'll need to drive change within your organization.

Sample Cultural/Education Assessment

Category	Question
Communication	What have you communicated to your team about this project so far?
	How has your team perceived this project (and the requirements it makes of them)?
	What communication vehicles do team members routinely use (list all):
	Telephone, E-mail, Voicemail, Video, Intranet, Newsletter, Other
	What type of communication seems to work best for team members? Have you launched a similar program in the past that had effective communication results?
	Do you have a web-conferencing tool in place?
Culture (change readiness)	What concerns, if any, have members of your team expressed regarding implementation of the EHR?
	What else is going on in the organization that might impact this initiative?
	What previous experience (positive or negative) has your team had with similar initiatives?
	Is there resistance or internal politics that should be considered?
	How will people's roles and responsibilities be impacted?
	What aspect of this initiative do you think your team fears most?
Skill Readiness	What computer skills do your team members possess?
	Desktop, Clinical applications, PDA
	What new skills (outside of EHR product training) will your team need to acquire to successfully use the system?
	Which processes/workflows will change with EHR implementation?
Training Delivery	How do you envision the training process?
	How has training been accomplished in the past?
	What sort of training do you think will be most effective for your team?
	What training expectations (i.e. mandatory/optional) will be shared with your team?
	What training time-commitment has been communicated to your team?
	Will you support required "self-study" in preparation for classroom training?
	Do you have a training facility (classroom) in place?
	When will a test system be available to "play" on?
Training Evaluation	How will you measure the success of training?
	Will you formally evaluate your team's understanding of the product (i.e. tests, certification)?

A sample cultural/educational assessment

Develop the Communication Plan

Once you've identified your executive sponsor and have completed the cultural/educational assessment, you're ready to formulate the communication plan. Chapter Six discussed the communication plan from the project team's perspective, focusing on keeping stakeholders (including users) informed of the implementation's progress. Here we'll touch on the topic again because good communication is key to assuring user acceptance of the EHR. If the material seems familiar, feel free to skip ahead to the next section.

A good communication plan should outline the process by which the organization will communicate to users the details of the EHR implementation—the "who, what, where, when, why and how" of it. Think about the last time your personal or professional life was impacted by a major change. The questions you had then are the same questions your users will ask:

- What exactly is happening? Give me the details.
- Why are we doing this? What is the benefit? What are the risks?
- When precisely will the change happen?
- How will my life change as a result of this?
- How can I best prepare for this change?

It's critical that your communication plan address these concerns. A.J. Schuler, Psy.D., an expert in leadership solutions and change management, advises that to win people's commitment for change, you must engage their interest on both a rational level and an emotional level. You can take Schuler's advice to heart by assuring that your communication plan addresses the emotional impact of the coming change as well as the facts behind it. As mentioned in Chapter Six, areas to cover in the plan include:

- Organizational Objectives: Explain the organization's overall objectives for the EHR. What does the organization hope to accomplish, and what are its deadlines for accomplishing it? How will success be measured and communicated?
- The organization's responsibilities and expectations: Explain the organization's responsibility for helping users prepare for change through education and ongoing support.
- The users' responsibilities and expectations: Explain what is expected of the users regarding time devoted to training and practice, and their responsibility for knowledge retention and evaluation.

- Personal Objectives: What's in it for me? Why would I, the user, want or need to use this system?

As you formulate the communication plan (see Appendix Three for a sample plan), remember that successful communication isn't a one-time event—it's a continuous process. The organization should measure and communicate progress on the EHR implementation on a regular basis. Consistent, timely communication helps maintain user support for the EHR. Conversely, inconsistent, or untimely information that's unskillfully presented can endanger user support for the implementation. And don't forget to regularly review your communication plan to assure your organization is sticking to it. When people are kept in the dark, they're more likely to create misinformation that's passed along through back channels or gossip.

What's Your Training Strategy?

Once you have established how you'll prepare your organization for change—through executive sponsorship, a cultural/educational assessment and the communication plan—you're ready to begin developing a training strategy. You'll begin by considering the results of the cultural and educational assessment that you conducted earlier. The assessment results will help determine how best to accomplish the key components of the training strategy:

- Who will conduct the training (internal resources vs. external resources, or a combination of the two)?
- When will the training take place (phased or all at once)?
- How will the training be delivered (classroom style, one-on-one, small groups, etc.)?

Who Will Do the Training?

The first step is to determine who will train your users—internal resources, the EHR vendor, or a third-party training organization. There are costs and benefits to all three options, so it's not a decision to make lightly. Issues to consider include cost, expertise, objectivity, authority, resources, and teaching tools.

VITALS

On average, successful software implementation projects allocate approximately 13% to 17% of their resources to human performance needs, such as change management, communication, education, training, and performance support.

Source: The Gartner Group

Internal Training

At first glance, using internal resources to conduct end-user training may seem to be the most effective method. Internal trainers have several advantages over outside experts: They're less expensive, more familiar with users' workflows and processes, and often have existing relationships with the users they are expected to train. Still, there may be risks to depending solely upon internal resources for training.

These risks may include:

- Lack of teaching experience. Can the internal trainers cater instruction to several different types of users? Physicians, for instance, have higher expectations of trainers than do front desk receptionists, so teaching them to use an EHR may require a highly experienced instructor who can adjust their teaching style appropriately. Physicians will rarely be able to devote more than a few hours to training, so the trainer must be able to provide just-in-time training quickly and effectively. Before deciding to use internal trainers, ask yourself whether your existing resources are capable of providing adequate training to the entire spectrum of users.

- Lack of motivation. Are the trainers themselves excited by the EHR and its great potential, or are they doing this because they have to? A highly motivated instructor produces motivated users; an indifferent instructor produces indifferent users.

- Lack of objectivity. Are the trainers able to visualize the improvements to their current workflows or situation without feeling defensive about the need for change? Clear vision is essential in someone who's introducing a disruptive new technology to potentially fearful users.

- Lack of authority. Will the users view the trainers as EHR experts? Since internal trainers rarely have working experience with an EHR, users are unlikely to recognize their authority to teach and thus may not cooperate or fully participate in the learning experience.

- Lack of resources. Are there enough internal trainers (and hours!) to conduct the end-user training within the designated time frame? Will their schedules be flexible enough to adjust to physicians' schedules (allowing for a blend of classroom and one-on-one training)?

- Lack of teaching tools. Can the internal trainers develop and/or customize appropriate teaching tools? After they leave the classroom, end-users are unlikely to be interested in using complex reference materials provided by the vendor, unless the materials are accompanied by clear, simple instructions.

Answer each of these questions honestly before deciding whether internal training resources alone will make your end-users comfortable and productive from day one.

Vendor Training

Many EHR vendors offer to conduct end-user training with their own highly experienced instructors. Just as with internal training, several factors will determine whether this training strategy is a good match for your organization.

- Cost. If vendor training is not included in your implementation costs, you may be charged additional fees. Compare these fees to the costs associated with pulling internal trainers from their normal positions.

- Training Experience. Trainers provided by the vendor are clearly experts on their own product but expertise doesn't necessarily make them good teachers. Ask them the same questions you would ask an internal trainer. Have they previously conducted end-user trainings? If so, was the organization similar to yours in size and composition? How many training sessions have they conducted before? How do they measure the effectiveness of their training? Are they available for follow-up contact after the training is completed?

- Familiarity with workflows. Does the vendor fully understand the organization's workflow and how users will employ the system? Do they grasp the intricacies of change within the organization, so that they can teach users how best to utilize the system?

- Objectivity/Authority. Trainers provided by the vendor will clearly be recognized as authorities on the product. And there is no question that they will focus on improving workflows and processes. But objectivity cuts

VITALS

Preparing training materials takes time. Based on our experience with training consultants, we recommend the following assumptions regarding development time for customization of training materials and classroom content:

- For each classroom hour of first-round training, eight hours of development time may be required. This 8:1 ratio (development to delivery) assumes minimal customization to existing, pre-developed training materials.
- If the training approach requires extensive updating of existing materials and the creation of additional training aids, then sixteen to twenty hours of development time per one hour of classroom time is a more realistic estimate.

both ways. Vendor trainers may be so excited about the EHR's benefits that they have difficulty empathizing with and addressing users' concerns about workflow changes.

- Resources. Does the vendor have the resources to train all of your end-users? The answer will depend on whether they normally provide training and thus are properly staffed. If they're not, the training they provide may pull resources from their implementation team, potentially delaying execution of the project plan.

- Teaching Tools. As we noted earlier, most vendors provide reference materials but not all provide teaching materials. Even if they do, the materials may not be customized to your workflows.

Third-Party Training

A third option to consider when developing your training strategy is to engage a training consultant. Looking back over the previous considerations, we can feel confident that training consultants are expert at training delivery, have the necessary objectivity, authority, and resources, and that they can build teaching tools customized for your workflow. The issues still left to consider are cost and expertise:

- Cost. Hiring a training consultant obviously costs money. However, a good training vendor can significantly speed up the training process and assure effective end-user utilization, thus paying for their services many times over. Questions to ask the training consultant include: Have they trained on this product before? What was the result? Do they have statistics regarding utilization following their training? Did the client re-engage them for follow-up training?

- Expertise. Again, it's important to consider whether or not the training consultants are expert in the product, as well as in your workflow. Have they conducted trainings on this product before? What type of training or certification did they receive on this product? Have they conducted trainings in a clinical setting? The consultants may be teaching experts, but if they don't thoroughly understand the product and clinical workflows, they may be a poor choice.

A Blended Approach

As we noted earlier, each of these three training strategies has unique costs and benefits. We recommend a blended approach to training that utilizes all three. Specifically, our experience has shown that the best training and utilization results are achieved when the following occurs:

- The vendor conducts initial project team training (discussed further in Chapter Ten) geared toward the people who will make design decisions about the EHR.
- Internal "super users" provide local support to their colleagues following training by third-party instructors. Super users are local experts in the product who understand clinical workflows and who've received some training in teaching methods and strategies. Though they are not necessarily responsible for end-user training, super-users support the training initiative and provide ongoing training and support to users as workflows evolve and the product is upgraded.
- A third-party training consultant is engaged to train the majority of end-users. The consultant organization must have experience creating, implementing and measuring the success of EHR training programs in clinical settings. We suggest you choose a training vendor that has an ongoing, close relationship with your EHR vendor. This helps ensure that the trainers are fully knowledgeable about the product and are directly supported by the vendor. Allscripts, for instance, has chosen The Abreon Group as their training partner. Before Abreon trainers become involved with Allscripts' clients, they must be fully certified on the products and agree to work closely with Allscripts' EHR experts to ensure quality of information and customer satisfaction.

VITALS: THE ROI OF TRAINING

Each one hour of end-user training provides five hours of value to the enterprise:

- Four hours of experimentation: An untrained end user may take up to 22.5 hours to achieve the same skill level that it takes a trained employee five hours to achieve (including training).
- One-half hour of help: End users require 0.5 hours less help from peers and centralized support desks for every hour of training they received vs. untrained end users' acquiring the same information.
- One half-hour of rework: End users spend 0.5 hours less time finding and correcting errors for every hour of training they received vs. untrained professionals performing comparable tasks.

Source: The Gartner Group

Of course, the cost of hiring a training consultant firm is not insubstantial. But since your organization has taken the initiative to implement a system of this importance, you should seriously consider the cost of *not* engaging training professionals (this is especially true for organizations working with an aggressive roll-out timeframe and many end-users). Such hidden costs include wasted time, wasted training effort, and increased end-user frustration and fear. Even if you have an internal education department, you should consider engaging the assistance of a training consulting group that is certified on the product, as their involvement in customizing teaching tools is extremely effective in driving and sustaining end-user education.

Planning the Curriculum

Once you've established (or at least considered) your training strategy, it's time to focus on the training curriculum. Experience teaches us that the most effective curriculum is one that's customized for the various end-user roles (providers, clinical users, non-clinical users, etc.) and focused on customized workflows (how end-users employ the product on the job). Such customized training is the most effective in producing high end-user confidence and utilization. In addition to being highly targeted, the curriculum should allow ample opportunity for hands-on practice in an applicable real-life scenario.

Developing a curriculum that's appropriate for your organization is not simply a matter of creating the right content and matching it to workflows. A complete curriculum must also consider *how* the training will be delivered throughout the organization. Depending on your organization's culture and educational readiness, you may choose one of four training delivery methods: the classroom approach, one-on-one training, self-study, or a blended approach.

Although each of these training methods can produce successful results, the best and most consistent results come from a curriculum that employs a blended approach. Because we all have different styles of learning, a blended approach assures that every user has the opportunity to learn and practice in a style that works for him or her, whether it is hands-on training or the study of reference materials.

A successful blended-training "flow" for an initial EHR implementation might look something like this:

• Assign Self-Study Classroom Preparation. Ideally, the training materials will be customized for particular end-user roles and workflows, and allow for some sort of self-evaluation and/or practice. Tracking of participation is critical to ensure success.

- Schedule Classroom or Small Group sessions. Instructor-led sessions, although logistically challenging, are the most direct method of assuring that users participate in the training, and that they understand the system and its workflows. Additionally, when they're appropriately conducted, instructor-led classes increase user confidence in their own abilities and in the organization's willingness to support the initiative.

- Use One-on-One Training in Select Cases: When classroom facilitation fails or evaluation results suggest that a user is struggling, one-on-one training (coaching) is usually the best alternative. Anecdotal evidence suggests that physicians who resist adopting an EHR are often won over by one-on-one training.

- Assess Users' Knowledge: Encourage training participants to complete a short exam following their training. The exams should take no more than 30 minutes to complete; include between five and 10 hands-on scenarios (one or two workflows); use multiple choice or true-false questions to test knowledge of general concepts; and require at least an 80-percent score to pass. You may decide that formal, scored exams will increase the level of fear among your users. In that case, we recommend that you continue testing for knowledge but without reporting the scores. Score reporting is less critical than the test's ability to spot users who require one-on-one training—as well as potential Super-Users.

- Provide Ongoing Support: Explain to training participants that educational support is always available, even after the classroom training is completed. Determine in advance how this support will be provided—will your IT Department be actively involved? For instance, during the implementation of the EHR at George Washington University Medical Faculty Associates (MFA) in Washington, D.C., the IT department dedicated a staffer to provide one-on-one training to every physician during their first "go-live" experience, just hours or days after they completed classroom training. Your organization may also consider establishing a "User Hot-Line" for a period of time (at MFA, they were able to discontinue the hot line two weeks after implementation). Quick reference guides are also valuable tools for continued user support. Again, identification of Super-Users is key, as they can help with additional mentoring or one-on-one training. Whatever ongoing support solution your organization deploys, communicate this to your end-users, so they won't feel abandoned after classroom training is complete.

Training Method	Description	Advantages	Disadvantages	Comments
Classroom	Pre-scheduled, "required" classroom attendance, facilitated by a trainer	-Tighter control of training -Consistency of training -Multiple trainees at once	-May not address different learning styles -Difficult to schedule -Difficult to enforce -May interfere with business operations	-Classroom sizes must be adjusted based on the level of training as well who's attending. -We recommend the following classroom sizes: Providers: small class sizes (3-4 physicians). Clinical Staff: Medium class size; up to 12 attendees with identical or similar roles Non-Clinical Users: Medium class size: Up to 12 attendees with identical or similar roles
One-on-One	Individual training of users by a trainer or Super-User	-Individual attention allows for flexibility in teaching styles -Assures that individual users clearly understand how to use the technology	-Expensive -Inefficient (only one user at a time) -May result in missed deadlines	One-on-One training may be appropriate for very small practices, or as a follow-up to classroom or small group training sessions where individual assessments suggest the need for additional focused time. This approach is especially well-suited to training physicians who resist new technology and/or refuse to attend classes.
Self-Study	Users are provided with appropriate training tools and allowed to study at their own pace, provided they meet established deadlines	-Inexpensive -Users can learn/practice at their own pace and on their own time	-Difficult to ensure compliance -May endanger project success if users aren't ready at rollout -Difficult to measure understanding	Appropriate for classroom preparation, as well as follow-up to retain comprehension. Must be accompanied by tracking reports and comprehension exams to ensure users are participating in the training and have the necessary knowledge.

Comparing Training Methods

Getting It All Done On Time

After getting this far, you might be forgiven for wondering whether end-user training requires its own project plan. The truth is, properly preparing for end-user training requires your organization to start thinking through the process and strategy long before the implementation begins. But don't despair. Help is available in the form of several useful planning tools. Below is a sample Training Project Plan checklist that can help you get it all done on schedule.

If this chapter has inspired you to begin a project plan with an end-user focus, then we've accomplished our objective. Remember, mission-critical projects that fail to live up to their potential usually lack a focus on the most important element—people. Best practices in an EHR implementation indicate that focusing on the end-user experience *before* go-live results in increased utilization and user acceptance. There's no better way to make end users comfortable and productive from day one.

Training Project Plan Checklist

Timeframe	Task	Comments
Upon contract signing	Identify Executive Sponsors and Change Leaders	
	Conduct Cultural/Educational Assessment	
	Develop Training Strategy	
Upon creation of Project Plan	Identify Training Resources	Get comfortable with the product and workflows; begin to develop training materials and plan classes
	Identify Trainees (roles)	
	Develop Curriculum(s)	
	Develop/customize Training Materials	Be sure to allow plenty of timefor this. (See inset for timing guidelines.)
4-6 weeks prior to Training	Build Training Schedule	
1-2 weeks prior to Training	Assign Pre-Work	
4 weeks prior to Go Live	Conduct Training	
4 weeks prior to Go Live	Prepare Ongoing/Support Training Resources	Advanced Users, Help Desk, Hotline, etc.
3 weeks prior to Go Live	Conduct Post-Training Knowledge Assessment	
2 weeks prior to Go Live	Practice in Test Environment	
1-2 weeks prior to Go Live	One-on-One Training (as necessary)	
	GO LIVE!	

Sample Training Project Plan Checklist

The Recap

- Communication, communication, and more communication! Spread the word throughout the organization to explain the what, when, why and how of the EHR implementation.

- Assess knowledge and provide basic computer skills as necessary. Demonstrate support and commitment to your users.

- Determine your training strategy. Don't overlook this in the budgeting process! Retaining a certified training group to drive the curriculum, create and customize materials, and to ensure end-user readiness may be the best investment you can make to ensure project success.

- Build your training project plan. The timing of your training must be in synch with your project plan, so start planning and resourcing immediately.

- Implement a support or follow-up plan. This can be as simple as identifying and publishing the names of your super users, or by following up with FAQs for a period following go-live.

If You Have Time

Creating Leadership Solutions for Profit and Growth, by A. J. Schuler, Psy. D. From "What's Up, Doc? Newsletter (September 2003). (http://www.ajschuler.com/What_s_Up_Doc_Schuler_Solutions_Newsletter_Sep_2003.pdf).

CHAPTER TEN

Assuring Quality and Operational Readiness

In This Chapter
- Get the right training for the project team
- Understand current and future workflow possibilities
- Keep the project on schedule and under budget
- Test the EHR software and validate the clinical data
- Formalize the vendor acceptance

Now that you've worked through the various issues of designing the project team, developing a training curriculum for users and generally setting the groundwork for the EHR implementation, it's time to test and evaluate the readiness of your new system prior to going live.

A few simple questions can tell you quickly where you stand. Have you developed a system for tracking every team member's progress in completing critical tasks on time? Have you prepared to test the system as you build it to assure the software configuration matches your intended workflow? Have you tested end-user acceptance of the new system? After you've completed several test cycles, are you prepared to review your workflow process and ensure it flows as expected? Finally, do you know how to provide formal acceptance to the vendor once the EHR is in production use?

If you found yourself hedging on the answers to any of these questions, then this chapter is for you. By the time we're done, you will have ensured that your team is not only ready to go but able to maintain its momentum throughout the arduous journey of an EHR implementation.

Training the Project Team

To truly assure the EHR's quality and operational readiness, start by providing the best possible training for the people who'll guide the implementation—the project team. Unlike end-user training (see Chapter Nine), the project team's training is provided by the EHR vendor alone and must occur *before* the design process and the majority of the implementation phase has been completed. The goal of training at this early stage is to boost the team's understanding of how the software works and how it can be manipulated to accommodate future workflows. Armed with that knowledge, the project team is better able to picture how each organizational role—nurse, physician, or billing clerk—will interact with the software.

The length of the training session will depend on the number of applications you've purchased. Training the team to use a complete EHR may take as long as one week. On the other hand, training for a smaller implementation of just a couple of modules could easily be completed in one day. Either way, training requires a big commitment of time that most busy professionals will resist. Whatever you do, don't let them talk their way out of taking part. It's essential that the entire project team complete the *full* training session to ensure that everyone is prepared to make the right choices about design and configuration. Nothing is more important to a successful implementation than good training.

Selecting the Trainees

If your EHR vendor hasn't limited the number of people who can attend the training, then every core project team member that can be spared should go. However, if the vendor has limited the number of attendees—or if your organization can't afford to lose the whole team for the duration—then make sure that at least one of each of the following is represented at the training session:

- The Physician Sponsor and at least one Physician Champion, if they are different (as Chapter Three outlines, the Physician Sponsor and all local Physician Champions also will attend a later, advanced training session intended only for physicians).
- The office manager
- The Project Manager
- The primary in-house trainer

These people, in turn, will be responsible for passing along their software knowledge to the remaining core project team members. This opportunity will enhance the initial trainees' knowledge of the application and ensure that everyone on the team is ready to make the fast-approaching tough choices about EHR configuration.

Preparing for Class

Now that you've chosen who will attend the training, assign them some reading so they show up prepared and familiar with the product. A well-prepared team lets the trainer focus on the details of the software rather than wasting time painting the big picture. The same process should be followed when the attendees return to train other members of the project team. Reading should include, at a minimum, all vendor website links including the company's vision and/or mission statement, the company history, any overview of software applications provided on the site, sales literature, news articles about the vendor and its products, and customer testimonials. Additional reading might include the vendor's reference manual, training manual and administrative setup guide.

After reading up on the vendor, carefully assimilate what you've learned about the company. What do they pride themselves on? What do independent journalists say about their products? What are they best known for? Are they a publicly traded company or privately owned? Who are their other customers and what do they have to say about the company? Knowing the answers to these questions will help the team build the close vendor relationship needed to support a successful implementation, not to mention ongoing operations after deployment.

Finally, everyone who attends the project-team training should clearly understand the role they will play on the team and what will be expected of them. Individual team members need to know how their contribution will affect the success of the project. Without this knowledge, it would be nearly impossible for team members to track and measure the quality of their contributions. To help clarify each team member's responsibilities, ask your vendor to provide a Resource Assignment Matrix that outlines the team's roles and deliverables (a sample matrix can be found in Appendix Four).

The matrix will require some time to develop, but it is a crucial team management tool that will come in handy later on.

Design and Build Activities

Design: The Big Picture

Now that the project team training has occurred, you're ready for the next phase in the implementation—designing and building. But before you can design the EHR you must clearly understand your organization's current workflows. What steps are taken when a patient calls the clinic to request a medication refill? Who takes the call? Where is it routed and how? How does the communication proceed? In the EHR design phase, these steps are called the "current state," or "current workflow." Working from the training your team has just received, determine how this medication refill request will be accomplished with the EHR. These new steps are called the "future-state workflows."

It's a good idea for your entire project team to fully engage in creating the future-state workflows. There are many ways to encourage their involvement but maybe the most effective is to first outline how tasks are performed today. Using sticky notes, write out the steps of a current sub-process, such as routing a patient's medication renewal request to a physician. Then post the sticky notes on a wall where they can easily be reshuffled to form a new workflow. Have the entire team participate so they can witness the workflow as it's being designed. With the software knowledge base that they acquired in training, the team can then translate the design into new steps to accomplish their joint goal.

This may sound like a cumbersome process but it's essential for two reasons. First, it's the best way to remove non-value-added steps in progressing toward an electronic workflow. Once all team members understand the existing process, it is easier to optimize the software's capabilities and to arrive at consensus. Remember, every team member brings their own unique experience to the table. When it comes to designing more efficient processes, it is extremely helpful to have someone from a non-related department who's removed from the daily grind to offer a non-biased opinion.

Second, the translation of current workflows into future-state workflows will help to identify training requirements for end-users. Understanding why a workflow was established in a certain manner is a great advantage for the training staff. As you read in Chapter Nine (Making Users Comfortable and Productive from Day One), the first step to take when training existing employees is to prepare them for change. Because employees don't always embrace change, and in fact may challenge training personnel in the classroom, it's helpful to understand the background of the workflows that they resist changing.

After you have transformed the current-workflow sticky notes on the wall into future-state workflows, you can translate them on paper using either an informal diagram structure or a software program such as Microsoft Visio. Once the design has taken form, share the hard copy with your vendor so they can verify the workflows prior to establishing the standard operating procedures. For additional information regarding the design portion of the implementation, see Chapter Eight (Going Paperless: Key Design Considerations).

Building a Better System

Design in hand, you're ready to begin building your EHR. The build process starts with setting up the software. Just like any other software program, the EHR lets you determine default settings, preferences or system options. If your team is responsible for defining the default settings, you will want to collect the list of preferences from your vendor (who will likely provide preferences for each application type, whether it's prescription writing, order entry, or charge entry). You can then assign team members to collect the data necessary to accurately define the preferences.

Completing the software setup may also include the task of data collection. For example, if a prescription-writing application will be utilized, you may need to load a list of pharmacies (names, addresses, fax and phone numbers) so physicians can fax them patient prescriptions. The vendor should be able to provide a comprehensive list of data elements that are needed and suggest ways to collect the data.

VITALS

Keep a diary of every system design decision and the intended result. This diary will ensure the system is set up as originally intended. For example, if you limited prescription writing to users who have a DEA number, but someone without a DEA is writing scripts, the diary will back up any corrective action you take.

With the design process underway, you can begin to think about end-user training. This assignment can be given to several team members, not just the trainers. For more details on end-user training, see Chapter Nine (Making Users Comfortable and Productive from Day One).

Finally, the team's clinical managers will have to create Standard Operating Procedure (SOP) manuals for employees. Unlike the training materials that explain how to accomplish tasks using the software, the SOP manual explains each employee's responsibilities for particular tasks. Many of these responsibilities may not be EHR-specific, so the SOP manual has a different but still important role to play within the entire change-management process. For example, an employee in the Medical Records department may be responsible for retrieving internal radiology films for patients, one day in advance of their appointments at an orthopedic clinic. Or a nurse may be responsible for calling pharmacies to verify their fax numbers when prescriptions fail to be sent using the number on file. The SOP manual will help ensure that existing and new employees alike understand how their jobs should be performed.

Defining Scope

As you prepare to test the software and its limitations, it's important to understand the project's scope. As described in Chapter Seven (The Project Manager's Role), the scope of a project explicitly states what is to be achieved and why it's necessary. For a project to be successful, the scope must be clearly recorded, understood, and agreed upon. If the scope is too vague, it's open to interpretation and invites the inclusion of redundant or excessive items in the project. If it's too strict, then the project may not deliver anything of real value.

It is far too easy to give in to pressures to exceed the project's scope and thereby place the implementation timeline at jeopardy. You say you'd never do such a thing? Well, consider the following situation. Let's assume you're implementing the EHR in a phased approach beginning with the prescription-writing utility. After three months the laboratory ordering utility is to be implemented. The scope document was written with this phased approach in mind and the future-state workflows specify that, for the first three months, lab orders will continue to be placed using pre-printed test order sheets that are hand-carried to the lab. However, one prominent physician member of the project team, who works in a very busy diabetes center, indicates he would like to immediately utilize both the prescription writing and lab order-entry utilities because doing so would save his department a lot of time. The system, he insists, will be of little benefit without both utilities.

So what should you do? First, take another look at the project scope. It clearly outlines the first-phase implementation of the prescription-writing utility, setting aside two months for implementation. Implementing lab order-entry at the same time would likely double the implementation time to four months. Such a drastic change is simply not acceptable according to the guidelines mutually agreed upon by the vendor and your organization's executive leaders. So the scope makes your decision easy. It also gives you the confidence you need to inform the well-intentioned physician that if he were to have his way the timeline of the entire project would be endangered.

In this and most other situations, knowing the project scope is essential to keeping the project on track.

Project Milestone Dates

To keep the implementation on target, the vendor project manager or your project manager (or both) typically creates a project plan using time-management software such as Microsoft Project or Excel. The plan will most likely include several milestone dates for "critical path" items—tasks so important that their timely completion is vital to bringing the project in on time and under budget. Every project team member should know all the critical path items and agree to immediately inform the rest of the team if their work threatens to place any of the critical path milestones at risk. Early warnings give the project managers time to come up with a back-up plan to get the project back on track.

How Is Your Team Doing?

One of the chief roles of the project manager is to keep track of team members' progress and assure that all critical path tasks are completed on time. A few simple steps can help:

- Organize weekly telephone meetings with the vendor's project team or project manager to ensure that everyone is progressing as expected. The meetings are also a good opportunity to discuss challenging workflows. Regular communication is also vital to ensuring that milestone dates are not pushed back.

- Organize regular internal meetings with the "builders" and remaining project team members. These meetings can be separate from the regular vendor meetings. Agenda items could include reviewing the progress of project team tasks outlined by the vendor; discussing how workflows should be defined; assessing progress on training materials; scheduling end-user training, etc. This again helps ensure that everyone is on schedule with their tasks and that the major milestone dates are intact.

- Establish, with the vendor's help, a methodology for team members to ask questions of the vendor or submit enhancement requests. The best mechanism may be a website, chat room, or better yet, an issue tracking system that all project team members can access throughout the implementation. Ask your vendor if they have such a system. Some vendors create a home-grown system, and others purchase one from another company. In any case, such a system allows you to login (and identify yourself as a customer), to view issues previously reported, and to view resolutions to those issues. Having such a central repository will prevent duplicate issue reporting and enable knowledge transfer for previously answered questions.

- Establish monthly executive meetings between the project managers and executive sponsors at your organization and the vendor. A high-level overview of the implementation project should be presented. This will highlight whether the project is on time and under budget, and enable the executives to assist in escalating issues when needed. Having no such forum could unnecessarily stall the implementation when conflicts cannot be resolved between your team and the vendor.

Test, Test, Test!

In the midst of building the system, the project team should be testing to ensure the software configuration meets the needs of your intended future-state workflows. Testing the software cannot be over-emphasized—it is *extremely* important. For example, try logging in as a physician and see whether you can prescribe medications. Can you prescribe all types of medications, including controlled substances? Log in as a front-desk clerk—are you limited to role-appropriate tasks or can you prescribe medications (hopefully not)? Can you log calls received from patients? Can you send electronic messages to physicians? Can you receive electronic messages from physicians?

The vendor typically has a list of steps they follow in testing the software after every upgrade or new feature release. Ask for the list and then expand upon it by including every possible user scenario that you can imagine. For help, look at training materials and the items from the diary that you kept during the build and configuration period. The diary should detail all the intended outcomes of every workflow as well as the intended outcomes of integration with third party systems. For example, if you were creating a test plan for prescription writing, you could list the steps required to prescribe a particular medication, but also indicate how to remove the medication if it was entered in error, or how to change the SIG after the prescription was already printed. The diary will raise important questions that will help you refine the testing process: If there are integration points with a practice management system (PMS) or ancillary systems, how should patient registration data be verified once entered in the PMS? Is the integration accomplished by a real-time connection or in batch mode (i.e., every night after midnight)? When should you see the update in the EHR? What subset of registration data can be viewed within the EHR? Are you receiving results from an ancillary system? What steps must be taken to get to that point? Who receives the notification that a result was sent?

During the testing phase, you may come across results that are different than you expected. Say, for example, that you're unable to fax a prescription for a controlled substance. The software will only print a hard copy for these prescriptions. You were under the impression that both controlled and non-controlled substances could be faxed. Some on your team may deem this a critical or "show-stopper" issue unless it's addressed. In this case, your project manager needs to evaluate, first, whether the unintended result is due simply to a misunderstanding of how the software works, or is the feature in question outside the project scope as it was originally defined? What are the consequences of dropping the feature? What are the costs associated with changing the scope (additional fees, extended implementation, increased internal resource costs) to include the feature? Is there a way to work around the issue and so avoid a project delay? For each such unexpected test result, review with the vendor and, if necessary, follow the proper escalation path to ensure that the team can proceed with the implementation.

Workflow Verification

Once you become more comfortable with the software through completion of several test cycles, you should be able to review your workflow process and ensure that it flows as expected. Separate the processes according to roles and verify with the appropriate project team member that there are no missing pieces. For example, are there any current processes for documentation that are not replaced by the EHR?

This is a good time for the project team to solicit feedback from end-users who have not yet been involved with the project. Select a small number of high-profile participants including physician sponsors and "super" users (for more information, see Chapter Seven, Building and Managing Effective Project Teams). Then use the training materials you've created to train the users, gaining valuable feedback on your training manuals and methodologies.

Time for a Dry Run

Now that the testing process is complete, it's time for a "dry run" of the software. There is nothing like simulating its use in the field with the users who will go live first. This is an opportunity for the hardware to be tested (printers, scanners, PCs, radio frequency network, PDAs, etc.) and for the users to once again verify the workflow, but now within their clinical environment. Most institutions run a simulation before each EHR module is implemented. Not all simulations should be run in the live environment of the clinic, however. The first simulation of your first module may need to occur with the vendor's supervision in a safe test environment like the one you used to solicit user feedback. Once you have a high level of confidence in the software and your users—typically after at least one simulation in a test setting—then you might decide to risk a dry run in the clinical setting. Even so, for your first clinical simulation it's a good idea to consider using test patients, just to reassure the users that their mistakes won't hurt anyone. If you're implementing a full EHR, then you may want to run two official simulation events for the first module—one in a test environment and the other in a live clinical setting.

It's a good idea to hold the dry run between two and four weeks prior to the go-live date. The timing is designed to ensure that you use the latest possible version of the software but also leave enough time afterwards to make any necessary adjustments. The selection of users for each dry run should include one or two physicians, their corresponding support staff (nurse, front desk, triage, technician) and a clinical manager. The showcase clinic or physician group should use the software continuously for at least a full day, preferably two, to realistically assess the new workflows and system configurations. Ideally, physicians and staff will accomplish this by utilizing "dual entry" of information (paper and electronic). This may highlight refinements in system configuration that can help end-users significantly when they use the software under higher-volume conditions. Another option is to choose a day when the physicians see patients in the morning and could devote the afternoon to the simulation, or vice versa. The staff members also must be available to implement their portion of the workflow process.

To ensure a successful dry run, some additional advanced planning is required:

- Ensure that all participants have completed a training session appropriate for their role.
- One day before the simulation, register all patients listed on the physicians' schedule and recreate their appointments so they appear within the test EHR exactly as they appear within the users' current system.
- Set up user login names, known passwords, and the appropriate security and access settings for all users participating in the simulation.
- Double check that all the hardware is ready for use and functional.
- If you are able to use the approach mentioned above of seeing real patients in the morning and simulating in the afternoon, then arrange ahead of time to have the morning's patient charts available for the physicians to refer to. This will help them remember their original assessments so they can accurately recreate the process with the EMR. The simulation then proceeds with the physicians repeating each patient's office visit but now using the EHR and its established workflows.

VITALS

Throw a bagel breakfast or pizza luncheon for participants in the dry run. For every hour of testing that users sit through, give them raffle tickets that can be exchanged for prizes (gift certificates, bonus vacation hours, items from your bookstore, etc.).

To include the support staff in the simulation, just run through each process as it would naturally occur without the EHR. Have one or more project team member act as "patients." Users should guide the patients through their workflows, following the SOP manual to ensure that every task they're expected to perform has been addressed either via the software workflow, through a revised paper process, or a combination of the two. The dry run should verify the established processes and ensure that the users and the hardware are all ready to go live.

Throughout this process, be sure the users have an easy mechanism for providing feedback. A good way to ensure feedback is collected is to assign two or more project team members to act as room monitors. They can walk around the room and answer questions, direct users when needed, and note when important issues arise. All feedback received from the users can help solidify your processes and ensure a smooth "go live" event.

After the simulation, call a meeting with the project team and the vendor to review the results. By now you will have answers to all the most important questions: Do any scenarios lack workflow processes? Did the users have questions about functionality that could not be answered? Was the level of training sufficient for users? Were there objections from the users that the team had not considered? After reviewing all the feedback, the team members may have to update the training materials, the training agenda, and the Standard Operating Procedure manual. If extensive changes are necessary, you may decide to hold another user testing session to assure that the changes produce the expected results.

Final Preparations

Now that testing and simulation has been completed, it's time to set up the live environment for production use. Some vendors may have computer utilities that copy the setup performed in the test environment. If so, use those utilities; if not, then ask your vendor for a checklist of setup items to ensure nothing is overlooked in this important step. Finally, once your live environment is set up for operations, it's important to run one last round of testing with test patients to ensure that everything runs smoothly.

> **VITALS**
>
> Celebrate the milestones you've achieved! And be sure to encourage your project manager and executive sponsor to verbally express their confidence in the team prior to going live. By now, every team member possesses the skills necessary to ensure a successful go-live event.

Providing Formal Acceptance

By this time, you've achieved many important milestones. Don't forget to celebrate your achievements! Of course, you still face many unknowns. Will the users be ready? Are they trained well enough? Is the E.H.R. ready? Did we think of everything? But consider that, after all the multiple iterations of testing you've performed, and the solid project team you will have on hand for the live event, you should be prepared to respond quickly to anything that comes your way.

But don't get too relaxed just yet. One additional process needs to be completed before you can sit back and celebrate. You need to provide formal acceptance to the vendor once the EHR is in production. The following checklist should be referred to throughout the implementation and will allow you to officially pronounce your acceptance upon live production use:

- Review the project scope (as outlined in Chapter Seven) and ensure that all noted items have been achieved
- Check that formal acceptance has been given to the vendor for each deliverable provided
- Check that all "show-stopper" issues have been addressed

If all of the above has been done, you'll be able to confidently sign the confirmation form signifying that the go-live goal has been achieved.

The Recap

- Carefully select the project team members who will participate in the vendor training.
- Ensure all project team members are prepared for their training by reading everything they can get their hands on in advance.
- Understand your current workflows—this will help you properly assess your organization's needs with the EHR.
- Carefully design your future-state workflows with the knowledge you have of the EHR. Use a whiteboard as you discuss each process that needs to be defined.
- Utilize the future-state workflows to create the end-user training materials.
- Keep a diary of every system design decision you make. This will provide you with both a checklist during your testing phase and a checklist as you move forward in building your live system.
- Create a Standard Operating Procedure (SOP) manual by utilizing the future-state workflows as a guide. This manual will help ensure that existing and new employees alike understand how their jobs should be performed.
- Understand the scope of the project. When testing the software, you will be less likely to veer off course if the scope is clearly defined.
- Utilize the dry run or simulation event to validate your future-state workflows, the SOP and the end-user training materials.

- Provide formal acceptance to the vendor once the software is in production use.

If You Have Time

- "Simulation Validation: A Confidence Assessment Methodology," Peter L Knepell & Deborah Arangno (www.iso.org).

CHAPTER ELEVEN

The Right Tool for the Job: The Critical Role of the IT Department

---

In This Chapter
- Inventory your environment
- Build in redundancy
- Create high availability and fault tolerance
- Avoid downtime
- Support end-users
- Make the system secure

If the transition to a paperless medical record is hard on doctors, nurses and administrators, for the much-maligned IT department it's something of a nightmare. Overnight, an electronic record adds a new mission-critical application to the IT environment. If the EHR operates as expected, it will radically improve the organization's efficiency and safety. But if it crashes, it can wreak havoc with patient care. And we all know who'll take the blame.

It stands to reason that the most important thing an IT department can do is to ensure the system's stability. Stabilization requires a wide variety of procedures, from analyzing the current hardware environment to taking steps to avoid downtime, reducing failure points and building in redundancy (translation for non-geeks: backing up). Once a stable hardware environment has been established to house the EHR, the next step is to support the application. Proper maintenance and monitoring will ensure that the EHR is running properly and prevent any foreseeable failures. And we can't forget the IT department's most public role—supporting the users through a help desk that's actually, well, helpful.

In this chapter we'll provide details on all of the above plus tips for developing organizational policies and procedures such as what to do in case of an unexpected system crash. It's the nuts and bolts chapter about the system's critical technology backbone.

Making the System Stable

The paper medical chart is one of the most vital forms of information at a healthcare organization because it houses all patient health information. The basic premise of the Electronic Medical Record is to remove the paper chart from your organization. This transition from a paper format to an electronic format places an enormous amount of responsibility on the IT department. You are adding a mission critical application to their environment, which can affect the entire organization if it fails. For this reason, the most important thing an IT department can do is to ensure that the EHR is stable and highly available.

It's hard enough convincing users to use a new technology that's stable; convincing them to use one that's constantly breaking down is nigh on impossible. It follows then that to generate confidence in the EHR and encourage its use, the system must first be made stable. The key implementation events that can help instill confidence in the new system are group training and the initial go-live. First impressions, as we all know, are the most important. Since most end-users will meet the EHR for the first time in the training room, it's important that this is a positive experience, rather than one that will reinforce potentially negative early impressions of the system (as Chapter 12 will point out, a major roadblock to EHR utilization is fear of new technologies and new ways of performing habitual tasks). Similarly, go-live is the first time that users will actually have to perform their jobs with the new application. It's a stressful time for everyone in the organization and also the best possible opportunity to build confidence in the system.

But first it has to be stable.

Understanding the Hardware Environment

There are many tricks to ensuring a system is stable. The first is to understand the environment that you are working with. If you are still in the decision making process, try to work with a vendor that supports technologies that are familiar to your staff. For instance, if your organization currently uses Oracle or SQL Server as database management software, try to find a vendor that supports that same application. In some cases it will be impossible to avoid new technologies, such as wireless networking or handheld devices, but minimizing the number of new technologies that need to be installed will dramatically reduce the IT workload.

One easy way to do this is to list all the technologies that the prospective EHR application uses and then determine if your team can support them all. If the EHR requires a higher level of technical skills than your team possesses, such as server administration techniques, then do your best to fill that need.

Another fairly simple part of understanding the hardware environment is to verify that the technologies required for the EHR will integrate into your current environment. For instance, if you're going to implement a Web-based application and your organization currently utilizes a proxy server, will the Web content work successfully with your current configuration? A proxy server can wreak havoc on a Web-based application due to blocked content or the caching capabilities of the device. You may need to upgrade or change the configuration of the server to get it to work with the EHR's Web applications. Catching similar conflicts early in the implementation process will ensure that you have a plan to resolve them before go-live.

VITALS: AN ENVIRONMENTAL CHECKLIST

- **What physical devices are part of the environment? (Include devices such as servers, hubs, switches, modems, VPN, access points, and printers).**
- **What services and software are required for the EHR to work properly?**

Simply outlining these basic requirements will give your organization a clear understanding of the pieces that need to be protected and managed.

Depending on the requirements of the EHR, your organization may need to make drastic modifications to the current infrastructure. For instance, if the EHR requires Microsoft's Active Directory to work properly, and your organization is still running an NT domain, you'll need to make major changes to your infrastructure to support that the new system. In most cases, the EHR will adapt to various infrastructures, but it's important to review this prior to making a purchase, or if that fails, very early in the implementation. Ask your vendor for a list of minimum specifications to ensure that you can easily meet them.

Besides analyzing your existing hardware environment for compatibility issues, it's important to understand the hardware environment that the EHR brings with it. It will most likely require multiple servers that perform different tasks. The EHR vendor should provide documentation and training regarding each of the servers in the EHR's environment. Be sure that you clearly understand each server's role and the function it provides. Some servers may be more crucial than others. For instance, a database server stores all information for an EHR. If that server has a failure, the entire system will go down, jeopardizing patient care. To avoid that nightmare scenario, you'll need to consider redundancy.

Building Redundancy and Fault Tolerance

Building in redundancy (commonly known as backing up your system) can be expensive. But not building it in—which is the same thing as not planning for system failures—is so dangerous as to be unthinkable. The unfortunate truth is that it is not a question of whether failures will occur but when. So the real question is, how will your organization deal with the failures you'll inevitably face?

Before we answer that question, let's consider why failures are inevitable. It comes down to complexity. Technologies like the EHR deliver immense benefits in the way of enhanced productivity, safety and financial returns, but accomplishing this requires an equally immense amount of complexity behind the scenes, powering the solution. The whole of any complex system is the sum of all its parts and their inter-dependencies. The key to building a stable system is to understand the possible failure points and the solutions available in these areas to guard against failure or quickly restore the system's availability. And the first step on this path is to build in redundancy.

Our experience has shown that most people choose not to look into redundancy initially because the cost seems excessive. After all, it's hard to understand why redundancy is needed—unless your organization has suffered the kind of massive breakdown that reveals the true magnitude of your danger. To illustrate this point, imagine what would happen if all of your paper charts were suddenly to vanish. Obviously, providers would have no way to access critical patient information. The situation is akin to a mechanic who's been stripped of all his tools. What's he supposed to do—kick the engine until it works? Of course, your paper charts are unlikely to suddenly vanish, but it could happen to your electronic charts—unless you build in redundancy.

Know the Price of Failure

To determine the magnitude of the risk you face, ask your clinical staff how their patient care would be affected if they couldn't access the patient charts for thirty minutes. For half an hour they may be able to complete their jobs by reverting to backup procedures, with little effect on patient care. But what if you extend the downtime to several hours or a day? The answers to two questions can tell you whether you need redundancy or not. How much downtime can you afford? And what price are you willing to pay for high availability?

Calculating the cost of downtime can be a difficult feat in itself, but it's not so hard to develop a fair estimate. First, outline all the tangible costs that would be affected by downtime such as employee costs, employee recovery costs, unexpected expenses, IT recovery costs, lost income, and value loss. We'll run through them one at a time:

- Employee costs refer to the hourly wage that is consumed during the downtime. For example, if your average employee makes $20 per hour, you have 100 employees and the downtime is an hour, that one hour will cost your organization $2,000 ($20 per hour x 100 employees = $2,000).

- Unexpected expenses occur when you must revert to backup methods. For instance, you may need to use prescription pads or paper forms that normally gather dust on a shelf somewhere. Replacing them is an unexpected cost.

- The next item is employee recovery costs. How long will it take employees to catch up from the downtime? Will employees have to input data that was collected manually during the failure? If the system went down for three hours, it may take an hour to recover. You may occasionally have to pay overtime or hire temporary workers to help make up the lost work time, so calculate that cost, as well.

- IT recovery costs are, obviously, costs incurred by the IT department, including time and any expenses needed to repair the system.

- Loss of income occurs when patient care is interrupted due to system downtime. For instance, a surgery may be scheduled that requires a physician to review a transcribed dictation that is only available electronically.

- If a patient develops a negative view of your organization because of the downtime, they may take their business elsewhere and encourage others to join them. This reduction in "perception value" ultimately affects your bottom line.

After estimating all of these costs, if you still determine that the initial cost of redundancy is more than your organization can afford, plan for it in the future. Make sure that the next application server you buy meets the requirements of a highly available system. For example, map out the redundancy technologies that you would like to utilize, such as clustering (we'll explain that in a minute) and ensure that the hardware supports it. Over time, this strategy will allow you to move to a redundant system without buying all-new hardware.

Help for Redundancy-Building

If you've decided that the risks of ignoring redundancy outweigh the costs of building it in, then you'll find that a variety of helpful redundancy-building technologies and techniques are available on the market. These technologies include clustering, load balancing, Redundant Arrays of Inexpensive Disks (RAID), and data replication. Clustering and load balancing are forms of server redundancy while RAID and replication are forms of data redundancy. Each of these solutions pursues a different path to achieving the same goal—ensuring that your system is always available to users, no matter what goes wrong.

VITALS: COMMON REDUNDANCY AND FAULT TOLERANCE TECHNIQUES

Clustering: Configures multiple servers to perform the same task.

Load Balancing: Evenly distributes the user load over multiple servers. Typically reserved for Web servers or application servers.

Redundant Array of Inexpensive Disks (RAID): Provides data redundancy by combining two or more mirrored hard drives to boost fault tolerance and performance, usually in servers.

In general, clustering is the way to build in redundancy for systems that store and manage data for end-users or applications. Examples of servers that would typically be used with clustering are file servers, print servers, and database servers. Load Balancing is generally used for application servers whose main job is to manage communications between end-users and a storage server. A Web server is a perfect example of a server that would normally use load balancing to add redundancy to an environment.

Avoiding Downtime Through Fault Tolerance

The EHR is going to become one of the most important applications in your environment. The safety of patients and the sanity of clinical users will depend on its smooth operation. For this reason, the system must be available as continuously as possible, to suit the 24-hour nature of medicine. And it must be able to handle failures without affecting the end-users—in other words, it must be fault tolerant.

Hardware or Software changes that don't go as planned are the number one cause of fault-related downtime. Relatively straightforward tasks such as upgrading an Operating System, adding disk space, or applying patches can all cause unexpected complications. Not every situation is avoidable, but with proper planning, many are. By following a few of the recommendations below, you can help avoid extended downtime:

• Change-control planning. Maintain a documented set of any changes being made to the system. Complete a full restart of the system at the time of the change to narrow the cause of an update gone awry.

• If you have the option to test a new software version or a new piece of hardware, by all means perform the available tests.

• Because even a minor update can cause unexpected downtime, plan for the system to be unavailable during the update.

• Give yourself time, when doing a system change, to make the change, test the change, and back it out, if necessary. If the change is to a critical component, such as a drive system or operating system, ensure that you can restore the system if the update doesn't go as planned.

• Complete backups that will allow you to recover the system from any state. It's also a good idea to have a redundant system that end-users can continue to work while the system is being restored.

The key to keeping things afloat in times of adversity is to build flexibility into your environment. Having options in place that reduce the chances of adversity triumphing will give you the edge to beat back the challenges and win the day.

Failing to Plan is Planning to Fail

After you've determined what hardware to implement, you must reduce as many single points of failure as you possibly can. Failure can occur on any device that's situated between the application and the client device. For example, a server with one network interface card (NIC) can introduce many points of failure. The NIC is connected to a Switch or Router with a network cable. The NIC, cable, Port, and Switch or Router all become a single point of failure. If you added another NIC card and plugged it into a second Switch, you will have eliminated those devices as single points of failure.

Evaluate your entire environment to map all possible points of failure. Once you have collected this data you can perform two important tasks. First, determine which single points of failure you can safely remove. For instance, if your servers are all plugged into the same Uninterruptible Power Supply (UPS), you could add another device to remove that single device as a failure point. This is the optimal choice, but it's not always possible. For the remaining points of failure, clearly document the process that needs to be performed to resolve an issue, if it should occur. Using the NIC example above, if it was found to be impossible to add a redundant NIC, you would outline a process for replacing the device. Having a process in place to resolve the issue if it does occur will reduce the amount of downtime you face, and lower the amount of stress during that period.

The same steps should be followed in creating disaster recovery procedures. Planning for disasters (natural, not man made) is the best thing that you can do. If something fails, you want to know exactly what steps you need to take to replace it, especially when your boss asks you how you are going to resolve the issue. When documenting disaster recovery procedures, it's also important to test them. This ensures that you have documented the process correctly and also allows you to practice. To help ensure that others can understand your procedures, other members of your team should practice disaster recovery as well. These documented processes should be easily accessible to everyone on your team in an electronic and paper format. Because the last thing you want to do on your vacation is talk someone through a recovery.

Supporting the Application

Establishing a stable hardware environment provides a solid foundation for the EHR to be housed on. The next step is to support the application. Luckily, this process is similar to supporting any enterprise application that you currently run. Proper maintenance and monitoring, including routine backup procedures, will ensure that the application is running properly and should prevent any foreseeable failures.

Backing Up

The most important aspect of an EHR is the data it houses. For that reason it's vital that you have proper backup procedures in place. A proper backup solution covers many things, not only the data you backup. There's the format of the backup, the safe storage of the information, and the ability to restore the information, as well—all key considerations.

It's important to understand exactly what data needs to be backed up and where clinical data is stored. At the very least you should ensure that clinical data is heavily protected so that you have little or no loss of data if a disaster occurs. But how far you go in protecting other data will play a big part in determining how long the system stays down after a disaster. If everything were destroyed except the clinical data in the EHR, you would need to manually restore all of the associated applications and hardware configurations, including the operating system, server configurations, and any applications that are required for the EHR to function properly. In the end you would get your system back up, but it could take entirely too long. And excessive downtime can cost lives in a medical setting.

For that reason it's preferable to complete full system backups every week and incremental backups periodically throughout the week based on your organization's requirements. In most cases, incremental backups happen each night. Regular incremental backups allow for faster backup because you're only gathering the data that has change since the previous backup. So the more often you backup, the less data you'll have to deal with during each backup. On the other hand, completing a full system backup every week gives you the data you'll need to restore the entire system at once, alleviating the need to manually install the operating system, supporting applications and system configuration. The full

> **VITALS: CHECKLIST FOR BACKUP POLICIES**
>
> To ensure that your backup procedures are complete, your policies should:
>
> - Define the level of backups that must be taken
> - List the backup techniques that should be used
> - Define what data needs to be backed up
> - Decide how long do backups need to be stored
> - State how many versions of the system should be stored
> - Define what data needs to be captured for backing up

system backup restores everything necessary for the server to become operational. For that reason, this method is much faster and can reduce downtime.

Backup Methods

Many methods exist for backing up data, including tape (a popular method), SAN devices that allow for data replication, or advanced database software that allows for log shipping—just to name a few. Whichever method you choose, the key is to understand the limitations of the solution so it doesn't become a crutch that keeps you from doing everything possible to ensure that your organization's data is complete and secure. Most organizations use enterprise solutions for backing up other applications. We recommended that the EHR be incorporated into that solution to ensure familiarity and to avoid adding more complexity to your environment.

If you don't currently have an enterprise backup solution, do your research and make sure that you choose a solution that will fulfill your organization's current and future needs. If you have twenty-five physicians and you expect to grow at a modest but steady rate, a tape solution would handle your needs far into the future. On the other hand, if you foresee massive growth in the near future, you should plan on incorporating other devices such as a SAN. A SAN device can handle up to a terabyte of storage (that's one-thousand gigabytes, or the equivalent of roughly fifty top-of-the-line computers). If your system requires 100 gigabytes of storage, and you're using a SAN, you could allocate a section of the terabyte to that system, then allocate another 100-gig section for replication of the original data. Having this copy of the data works as a backup solution and the partitions can be reassigned. Which means that if the original drives fail, you can quickly point the server to the replicated data, enabling swift recovery.

Rotating the Data

Once the data is completely backed up to a device, it's vital that it's kept safe and protected from every possible threat, human and natural. The best "rotation" includes an off-site storage location that is fireproof and waterproof. Proper rotation means exactly that—rotating the various sources of backup data to ensure that you have as many up-to-date versions of the application as possible. If an event occurs that corrupts data, you need to be able to restore to a point in time prior to that the most recent backup. Rotating the tape allows you to restore to any point necessary.

Confused? Let's look at an example. Imagine that you completed a system backup last night. Previously that evening, one of your associates mistakenly made a change to the system that incorrectly files data. The bad data goes unnoticed until the following morning when a nurse catches the error. At that point your team determines that there is no way to identify the corrupt data and most importantly, there is no way to correct it even if you could identify it. Now, if your latest version of the system backup was from the night before the change, you could easily revert back to that version. So having multiple versions of the backups allows you more flexibility with your restoration options.

The Disaster Recovery Plan

The last step in backing up the system involves ensuring that you can restore the system from the information that you've backed up. Many organizations run their restoration process for the first time only after a failure occurs—a questionable strategy at best. If your job is to ensure the safety of all data stored on a device, and the system has a complete failure, how sure are you that your device contains all the backup data you'll need to restore? Would you stake your job on it? No? Then your team had better develop a disaster recovery plan and get to work testing it.

Disaster recovery plans can be extremely elaborate, but all successful ones are based on the premise that you have successfully backed up the right data, you have defined and tested the steps necessary to recover the data and the system, and you have the proper resources available and in place to perform these functions. In general, then, the disaster recovery plan should include the exact steps that need to be taken to complete a full recovery. These steps should be practiced repeatedly until your entire team is comfortable completing them. Practicing your response to a data disaster ensures that you have everything you need to easily handle the restoration.

Maintaining the System's Health

If you suddenly developed a fever and a sore throat, you might guess that you were coming down with the flu. The symptoms are a warning to expect illness; if you catch it early enough, you might be able to get enough rest to stay healthy.

Believe it or not, a server operates in the same way. Before a failure occurs, symptoms of the upcoming crash will begin to surface. But you'll only spot the symptoms if you have been actively monitoring the system. The most common items to monitor are the various system logs. Typically, an operating system has a log that applications write events to. For instance, Microsoft has the Event Viewer that allows you to review application, system, and security logs. Reviewing these logs on a regular basis will help you become familiar with normal events and easily pick out events that require your attention.

Monitoring techniques vary based on the applications in use and the operating system that's being utilized. Most applications have built-in monitoring tools or automatically recommend actions to take to ensure that the system is in good health. Completing these steps will help reduce failures and increase the availability of the system.

Capacity Planning

The final consideration in supporting the application is capacity planning—making sure you have enough storage space for your data. Most vendors will provide guidelines for maintaining the capacity necessary to support future growth, but don't rely entirely on the vendor. Because universal guidelines don't apply to every environment, it's important to track your capacity needs internally.

Fortunately, storage consumption is one of the easiest things to track. During the implementation the system will have huge spikes in growth initially due to system setup and data conversions, but over time you should be able to get an idea of the growth trend. It's important to take these measurements periodically to plan for future growth. If you currently have fifty gigabytes available in your system and you normally grow at a rate of ten gigabytes per month, it's pretty easy to determine that you will need more drive space within the next five months. Which, by the way, doesn't mean that you can put off the planning for five months. It's much easier to plan for growth when you have time than to wait until the day you run out of space.

The same is true for system resources. There are many resources to monitor, such as memory utilization and processor utilization. These resources are usually spot-checked periodically throughout the week, preferably at different times of the day. It's important to fluctuate the time when you capture these measurements to ensure that you spot different levels of activity on the system. The measurements also ensure that the hardware can handle the load that the application is placing on it, and plot trends for the necessity of future upgrades.

Manually monitoring your logs can be a time consuming task. Many third-party applications can complete most or all of the steps required for proper system maintenance, as well as monitoring the system 24 hours a day. In most cases the tools will alert your team of an issue before an end-user even notices there's a problem. They can also be used to take an action if specific failures are found. For instance, if a vital service is stopped, these tools will attempt to re-start them. In some cases, the issue may be resolved without human intervention. The basic premise of these applications is to ensure that proper monitoring occurs in the background and that the system remains healthy.

VITALS

Third-party monitoring and maintenance tools can spot problems before you do ... and fix them without human intervention. Some popular applications include:

- IPSentry
  (http://www.ipsentry.com/)
- WebTrends
  (http://www.netiq.com/
  webtrends/default.asp)
- ipMonitor
  (http://www.ipmonitor.com/)
- OpenView
  (http://www.management
  software.hp.com/)

The system resource trends that you measure can also be important during application upgrades. As new technologies are adopted, your system resources may be stretched to their limits. For instance, an upgrade may incorporate biometrics into the applications' user-authentication process. This new technology may add extra stress to a server that was never intended to handle biometrics. . To ensure that new requirements don't interfere with system performance, it's important to test any new technologies before bringing them live.

Selecting the Right Device for the Job

Selecting the right device is one of the most important decisions to be made in an implementation. With any job, the tools craftsmen use can have a huge impact on the outcome. Would you use a wrench to pound in a nail? It might work but it's inefficient and impractical. A hammer works much better. To determine which devices are appropriate for the many different requirements of the EHR (should doctors have PDAs or desktop PCs, or both?) you not only have to understand the hardware environment that you're implementing in—you also have to know your end-users and understand their needs.

To help with this task, try mapping out the groups that need access to the system and define their roles within your organization. Once you know who they are, determine the physical location from which the various end-users will need to access the system. Nurses may need access in the exam room or at the nurse's station but they're unlikely to access the system from home. Physicians, on the other hand, will enjoy the fact that they can access a patient's chart from home when they're paged at two o'clock in the morning.

Next, determine what information the different users need access to. A key advantage of an EHR is the ability to portion out information based upon the end-user's role. If the front desk staff doesn't need access to patient records, for instance, then you can block them from accessing this information.

Bear in mind, though, that there's a fine line between restricting access to a patient's record and preventing someone from doing their job. For that reason, it's imperative that this process be outlined and tested. After you've designed and built the system, you must perform simulation tests. This is accomplished by documenting each role's current workflows, translating them into future workflows and then following that design. (For a more detailed discussion of workflow design, see Chapter Eight).

All of this information will be helpful in determining which tools you can use for your implementation. Take what you've learned from assessing end-users' needs and apply it to the hardware. Compare the devices that you currently

User Role	Access Required
Physician/Nurse Pract	All – Full Patient Records, Schedules, Tasks, Billing Information
Nurse/Med Assistant	All – Full Patient Records, Schedules, Tasks, Billing Information
Phone Triage Nurse	Patient Demographics, Tasks
Other Clinical Staff (Lab techs, Rad techs, etc)	Patient Records, Tasks
Front Desk	Patient Demographics, Schedules
Billing Office	Billing Information
Medical Records	Partial Patient Charts
Transcriptionists	Patient Demographics, Partial Patient Chart
System Administrators	Full Access

An inventory of end-user access requirements

have deployed with your vendor's list of supported devices. In most cases those device may be a perfect fit. If you have determined that a physician needs access from anywhere, a desktop PC isn't going to work very well. There may be one device that meets all needs for a group, or it may take multiple devices. In either case, it's worth taking time to evaluate the available options.

Always seek end-user's feedback on your device decisions. Feedback is usually solicited fairly early in the implementation, because it's important that users become familiar with the system and understand how it works with the device. If you force something upon them, they may be reluctant to adopt the new device. If they are part of the decision making process, however, they will feel they have ownership in the decision and are therefore more likely to adopt.

Know the Value of a Good Device

It's also a good idea to evaluate the value the device is providing. Purchasing new equipment is often a large investment. Is the access that the device provides worth that cost? There are many options available to help reduce the cost. Leasing equipment can be an attractive alternative. It lowers the initial investment and can also provide future upgrade paths to new devices.

In some cases you may determine that a device is not worth the cost. For instance, your organization may decide that it's only essential to access the system from the office. Physicians may want access from anywhere, but the cost of the device is too much for your current budget. It may be a good idea to implement a program whereby your organization incurs some of the cost if a physician decides to buy the device. This will increase adoption with a lower cost to your organization.

Mobile devices often present technological challenges that your organization hasn't faced before. If the device requires network access you must ensure that access is available wherever the device will be used. This may require implementing a wireless network, which would require you to purchase access points and install wiring in the proper locations. To ensure proper coverage of the wireless network, a site survey should also be conducted. This survey ensures that the wireless connection will be available throughout the required areas and that the devices are properly configured. Mobile devices also usually have power constraints that aren't found in most other devices. It may be necessary to have power cords throughout the organization to recharge the devices if the battery life is shorter that the user's workflow.

Mobile devices also are harder for the IT department to manage. A normal PC is relatively easy to manage because it's always on the network in a stationary position. The worst case is that you need to walk over to it and apply the updates. But a mobile device can be virtually anywhere. The device could be in a physician's pocket, forgotten in an exam room, in a locked desk drawer, in a car, or even at home. This can make tracking down the device for updates difficult and time consuming.

It's also harder to ensure that the data is secure on a mobile device. If a physician leaves a handheld device in the exam room and someone steals it, how confident are you that there is no confidential data on the device? It's important to ensure that the device stores patient data in an encrypted format and that it requires authentication to operate.

Mobile devices are also easier to damage, lose, or forget. Your organization will need to ensure that ownership is pushed onto the physicians to ensure that they keep track of their devices. Some organizations require deposits or ask physicians to sign agreements stating that they will replace the device if anything happens to it.

Overall, mobile devices can be cumbersome to manage, but the benefits are well worth it. Having the ability to access patient data from virtually anywhere is an amazing benefit that can significantly enhance physician satisfaction as well as quality of care.

Supporting the End-Users

Implementing an EHR can be a burden for the IT department, and it places similar stress on the end-users. For most of them, the EHR will introduce entirely new processes. Imagine showing up at work tomorrow to discover that your entire way of doing things has been altered by a strange new technology. That's essentially the situation that your end-users will find themselves in throughout the implementation of an EHR (though the strain can be greatly mitigated by proper training and communication).

As a general rule, people don't like change. Some people will respond with optimism and may even love that they are learning new and better ways to do their jobs. But these folks are definitely in the minority. For the majority of end-users, the EHR implementation will be a real challenge. Helping them through the transition following go-live is the job of the help desk—the nerve center of the IT Department's outreach to end-users.

The Help Desk

Help desks exist for one purpose, to help end-users. The ultimate goal of a help desk is to ensure that technology within the organization is being used efficiently. The best way to do that is to help the end-users—and do it quickly.

Implementing an EHR will inevitably increase the volume of issues your help desk must respond to. For physicians and their support staff, the EHR will become one of their most heavily used applications. Prior to the EHR, it was the responsibility of different teams, such as medical records, to handle problems related to these workflows. Now, when a physician has trouble entering data in a patient's medical record, it's the IT Department's problem.

Fortunately, the increased burden on the help desk can be handled without hiring hoards of tech support personnel. The answer lies

> **VITALS**
>
> An important part of end-user support is answering their questions. Formats for doing so include:
>
> - IT Help Desk
> - Weekly "lessons learned" luncheons for end-users to share their stories
> - A FAQ database or knowledgebase
> - Vendor Help files that can be accessed via the software application
>
> Regardless of the format chosen, it's important to provide a high level of attention to users for the first month or two after the initial go-live. Keep them enthusiastic about using the EHR, and try to keep them from becoming frustrated, because frustrated users can quickly become non-users.

with the EHR "super users" who work at each location where the system is rolled out. Super users can quickly become the first line of troubleshooting—dramatically reducing the number of issues reported to the help desk. They possess a high-level understanding of the EHR and most likely were involved in the system's design. Even if they can't resolve the issue themselves, they'll likely know what next steps should be taken.

Help desks vary in formats throughout the industry, but the basic idea is to provide consistent, fast resolution to the end-users. It can take many attempts at providing great support, but the key is to continually make improvements based on end-user suggestions.

One example of a successful help desk format can be found at Cooper Clinic, a multi-specialty physicians practice with locations spread throughout northwestern Arkansas and eastern Oklahoma. Cooper has 129 physicians and more than 600 support staff but just five support technicians. This may seem like an overwhelming responsibility for the IT department, but through the use of an efficient and structured support model, they provide excellent service.

Doyle Reeves, Cooper's director of communications, explains the format of their help desk:

"We have a help desk center that is shaped to maximize efficiency. The area has two workstations, each with the necessary monitoring programs installed for redundancy in case of failure. The workstations have flat-panel monitors extended to allow the monitoring software to be viewable at all times. In most cases, problems are detected and corrected before end-users even notice. Applications send alerts to us via e-mail with audible notifications. Four technicians man the help desk on a weekly rotation, with the lead technician stationed nearby.

"Every device in our clinics has a label displaying the help desk phone number and e-mail address. Our help desk management software ties into Active Directory, has knowledge base capabilities, and links to our Intranet, so it gives users the ability to enter and view the progress of any incidents they report. Users can rate our service performance and the Intranet site also provides some useful documentation. Our service level agreement is posted online, as well as our incident-rating policies. We have a five-level rating system, Level One being the highest priority and five the lowest. We have departmental policies in place to dictate how we respond to the different levels. For instance, support staff is notified immediately for a Level One issue, with continuing updates on the hour. There's also a visual message board where the incident is displayed to notify everyone that a Level One issue is present. Technicians can view and close incident tickets from any workstation or from their PDAs.

"The help desk is also the focal point for vendor contact in most cases. If a call is entered with a vendor, their updates and responses are made through the help desk personnel, who pass the communications back and forth between end-users and the vendor. So when a physician calls in for a progress update on an issue, the help desk has the knowledge it needs to answer them. This reassures users that we know what we're doing.

"Technicians also have cell phones for communicating, as well as network paging software which sends text messages to dispatch them. All applications have assigned primary and secondary technicians. Since the person manning the help desk is a technician rotating in from the field, they have the experience to handle most issues immediately themselves."

Whether Cooper Clinic's help desk solution works for your organization or not, their example illustrates the flexibility and productivity that can be achieved through solid coordination and the creative use of available technology.

Securing Your System: The HIPAA Security Rule

The Health Insurance Portability and Accountability Act (HIPAA) of 1996 is a federal law that mandates a wide variety of activities for healthcare organizations large and small. You're probably already familiar with the difficult requirements of HIPAA's Transactions Standard but here we'll discuss only the Privacy Rule (effective April 14, 2003) and the HIPAA Security Rule (effective April 21, 2005, or April 21, 2006 for small healthcare organizations with receipts of $5 million or less). The HIPAA Privacy Rule pertains to all forms of protected health information (PHI), whether paper or electronic, and specifies the manner in which this patient data can be used. The Security Rule applies to PHI in electronic format only and is intended to ensure that the information is kept confidential and secure from unauthorized use.

For organizations that store all of their patient charts in folders in the chart room, security is a simple matter of preventing unauthorized people from removing the charts. In these organizations, the IT group is not concerned with who is allowed to request a chart and who isn't, nor is the group responsible for securing the chart room. But if that organization chooses to implement an EHR, its IT department will suddenly move to front and center in the battle to secure patient information. In addition to its current workload, the department will be asked to ensure the security of confidential patient data and comply with HIPAA regulations. While the EHR typically will come with a limited form of built-in security, securing patients' data is ultimately the organization's legal responsibility, not the vendor's. That's because HIPAA does not consider vendors to be "covered entities" that must abide by the rule. Therefore, it's important to have a firm grasp on where the application's security ends and your role begins.

There are many ways to understand security, but an important overall distinction to know is the difference between encryption (privacy) and authentication ("are you who you say you are?"). Encryption refers to the protection of data from prying eyes—it's the 'code' language that parents use around their kids when they want to keep a matter private. Authentication is the process of proving identity - the TSA officer at the airport checking ID's.

One frustrating truth about security is that there is no single solution that will make your information 100 percent secure. How can you be protected from threats that you cannot even imagine? Still, there are steps you can take to make your organization as secure as possible, even if you don't know what you're securing it *from*.

To effectively address security at your organization, consider the following strategies:

- Assign security to one person. Begin by looking at security management as a top-down process. HIPAA requires healthcare organizations to name a security officer as the point person for implementing the regulations. The security officer's charge is to oversee a formal security program, which includes conducting a risk analysis, creating procedures and policies, training employees, and maintaining deterrence. Another responsibility of the security officer is to ensure that all computers are kept up to date with security patches from Microsoft, and with antivirus and anti-spyware software. Be sure that it's set to automatically update the most current settings on a daily basis.

- Honestly assess the risks you face. HIPAA requires healthcare organizations to conduct a formal risk analysis as a first step to developing a security program. A basic risk analysis consists of asking yourself common-sense questions about how you and your staff currently handle HIPAA-protected health information (PHI). Even if you think you're not transmitting PHI electronically, the risk-analysis may turn up things you didn't realize you were doing. It's important to conduct risk assessment on a regular schedule because in addition to new threats being released on a weekly if not daily basis, the makeup of your organization will change due to employee turnover, new vendors and new technology,

- Develop a policy. Once you've assessed where and how your organization transmits PHI, you can develop a comprehensive security policy that outlines specific procedures your staff must follow to protect patient data. Guides to developing policies and procedures for the HIPAA Security Rule are available from the American Hospital Association, the American Medical Association, and other physicians' and institutional associations, as well as state organizations such as CAL HIPAA (www.calhipaa.com).

- Sanction violators. Perhaps the biggest security threat healthcare organizations face is from insiders—former or current employees who commit embezzlement or some other crime, or just someone who makes a mistake. Deterrence is key to preventing security lapses by insiders. Sanctions for violating the security policy can escalate from verbal warnings to written warnings to unpaid suspensions to firing.

As new vulnerabilities are discovered on almost a daily basis, it's important to stay informed about new security threats. Sign up with your security vendors to receive email alerts as these new threats are discovered.

Security Overview

- Ask your current vendors about the level of security they provide. Modern operating systems and many Internet service providers (ISPs) come with strong security measures built in.

- Carefully assess the real security risks that you face. A good risk-analysis will turn up things you didn't realize you were doing—and it's required by HIPAA.

- Develop a security policy that outlines specific procedures your staff must follow to protect patient data.

- Apply sanctions to anyone who violates the security policy. Deterrence is key to preventing security lapses by insiders, who pose perhaps the biggest security threat practices face.

- Back up your computer systems. HIPAA requires a contingency plan in the case of a computer crash, and it's only common sense to have a sound, automatic back-up program in place.

- Keep all computers updated with security patches from Microsoft, and with antivirus and anti-spyware software that's set to automatically update the most current settings on a daily basis.

The Recap

- Understand the environment. Knowing the technologies being implemented will ensure that your team has the technical acumen to support the environment and successfully migrate the EHR into your current environment.

- Maintain high availability and fault tolerance. End-users are going to expect this system to be available at all times. Determine what steps your team can take to ensure the system is available.

- Avoid downtime. Identify all single points of failure in your environment. Create plans regarding the steps necessary to resolve any point of failure. If possible, remove the single point of failure by adding redundancy to the environment.

- Build Backup and recovery capabilities. There is nothing more important than good backups. If disaster does occur, ensure that your team can recover from it. Failing to plan is planning to fail.

- Pick the right end-user device. Get user feedback regarding the different types of media available. Provide them with the tools to do their jobs where and when they need access to the system. Getting the users involved in this process will also give them a sense of buy-in and help increase utilization.

- Develop policies and procedures. What will your employee do during a failure in your absence? Defining clear policies and procedures will ensure that they have guidelines to follow during times of doubt. Continue developing these throughout the use of the EHR to ensure that they are kept up to date and that you've encompassed all possible scenarios.

- Support your end-users. Providing a stable system is only one piece of ensuring your end-users are going to successfully adapt to the EHR. Providing them with high-quality, timely support can also increase satisfaction and utilization.

- Conduct a risk analysis. There are many tangible and intangible costs to downtime. Determine what these costs are and how much downtime you can afford. The answer will determine what your budget should be for high availability and redundancy efforts.

- Maintain security. No single application can secure your environment from all possible attacks. Your organization should be actively looking for new ways to guard the environment against possible attacks, without making the system so secure that it restricts usability.

If You Have Time

- Windows 2000 & Windows Server 2003 Clustering & Load Balancing by Robert Shimonski. McGraw-Hill Osborne Media (April 9, 2003).

- Disaster Recovery Planning: Strategies for Protecting Critical Information Assets by Jon William Toigo, Jon Toigo. Prentice Hall (August 27, 2002).

- Computer Security by Dieter Gollmann. John Wiley & Sons (February 16, 1999).

- 802.11 Wireless Networks: The Definitive Guide (O'Reilly Networking) by Matthew Gast, Matthew S. Gast. O'Reilly (April 2002).

- Medical Privacy—National Standards to Protect the Privacy of Personal Health Information (HIPAA educational materials). http://www.hhs.gov/ocr/hipaa/assist.html

Portions of this chapter appeared in similar form in the article "Hack Attack: How Safe Are Your Computers?" Todd Stein. Physicians Practice (February 2005).

CHAPTER TWELVE

Utilization Management: Strategies from the Real World

In This Chapter
- Utilization management and why it's important
- Seven principles of EHR utilization management
- Build a UM program
- Strategies from the real world
- Overcoming perceived roadblocks

If the previous chapters share one message, it's that giving the green light to an electronic health record is only the first milestone on the EHR journey. The most sophisticated and elegant of EHRs is but a bright promise until it is fully functional and its users are appropriately trained. And even then there's no guarantee the new system will be widely used. In fact, the truly complete EHR can only be achieved by a deployment program that's designed around the principles of utilization management.

Utilization management is the bridge from the dream of an electronic record to its reality. By working with the product vendor, the footings can be laid, the towers raised, the cables strung, the roadway built and test vehicles driven across. But getting the users to cross the bridge is still not automatic. The situation is akin to the early days of large suspension bridges, when many people feared making the crossing and had to be driven across or advised to take the local ferry. In many respects, we're still at that point today with the EHR.

In this chapter we'll tell you how to build a successful utilization program, and guide you through a variety of common problems. Rather than repeat a set of textbook principles, we'll present strategies that have worked in the real world by reviewing the results of 20 EHR implementations, both failed and successful. Our intention is to convince you that utilization management is a science with precise, disciplined methods. If you'd prefer to hear the usual message of magic bullets and wishful thinking, you've come to the wrong place. But if you want to know how to get your doctors to use that new EHR you invested so much time and money in, read on.

What Is Utilization Management and Why Is it Important?

Few people would buy a new home but refuse to use the heating system just because it had computerized controls. Similarly, it would seem strange, even unprofessional, to buy a new and proven medical technology but use it only half the time, or with half the patients who could benefit. Yet that is exactly the situation faced by healthcare organizations after implementing an electronic health record. Despite the organization's best efforts to encourage utilization, many doctors simply will refuse to use some or all of their new EHR's functions.

Why is it that partial usage of an EHR is acceptable in healthcare while the refusal to use mission-critical technology in other industries would not be tolerated? Why is this situation allowed to persist despite the vast amount of money, time, and other resources invested in EHRs? Why isn't full utilization the assumption of every implementation?

What's wrong with healthcare, anyway?

Hyperbole aside, the answer is fairly simple. EHR utilization programs don't fail from lack of trying but from a lack of empirically driven methods. One example is the widespread assumption that IT staffers should be the evangelists of utilization, despite years of empirical evidence suggesting that physicians trust only their peers' advice on technology issues. Another indication that empirical methods are missing from utilization management is the common assumption that a good implementation plan will ensure utilization. That could not be further from the truth. Utilization can be improved and operational efficiencies can be attained even after the implementation has been completed.

Best-practice organizations realize early on that utilization management must be a deliberate, strategic process if the EHR is to achieve its expected outcomes. They also realize that it really is not about technology, but about helping providers to transition to a new set of tools. Thanks to their hard work and perseverance, lessons from the field are beginning to build a true science of repeatable methods that can be employed anywhere with similar results.

The Seven Principles of EHR Utilization Management

From our observations of EHR implementations—the successful ones and the less successful—we've distilled seven key principles of utilization management. We believe organizations must have a basic understanding of these principles if they hope to achieve their EHR utilization goals.

1. Success begins and ends with physicians
2. Utilization must stay on the leadership's radar
3. High utilization targets promote high utilization
4. Experience is the best teacher
5. Theories are only as good as their results
6. Utilization promotion only works if you work it
7. Financial incentives aren't magic bullets

Principle One: Success Begins and Ends With Physicians

By now, you should be familiar with this book's guiding principle: If Doctors Don't Use It, Nothing Else Matters (IDDUINEM). Because physicians are the beginning and the end of utilization management, it pays to understand their mentality. Physicians enjoy a justifiably high standing in society, but in at least one way they are just like everyone else. Before they'll do what you want them to do, they have to know that you empathize with their needs.

To garner their respect and support for your project, you must provide physicians with a support system that respects their profession, practice, constraints, and schedules. In this effort, one-on-one training and on-site, personalized support is a great help. In general, as we have

VITALS

At Affinity Health Group, a 27-physician multi-specialty practice in Tifton, Georgia, the Physician Sponsor held weekly lunch meetings during and after the practice's EHR implementation (with food provided by pharmaceutical reps). The popular meetings became peer training sessions, allowing physicians to ask other physicians basic technology questions.

outlined in Chapter Three, you should take pains to involve your organization's physicians in every step along the implementation path, and make sure that their concerns have been addressed before moving on to the next step.

Principle Two: Utilization must stay on the Leadership's Radar

Utilization management kicks into high gear only *after* the EHR has been deployed, not before. That's because human nature will lead the system's users to gradually slip back into habitual ways of doing things, once the spotlight has strayed from implementation and meeting the initial utilization targets. To attain high levels of utilization, the topic must continually come up for review. In the early stages it's fine to initiate temporary measures, such as assigning support staff individually to end-users. Eventually, though, the end-user community must sustain their own utilization largely unaided—except for the urging of management. Revisiting utilization on a regular basis in leadership meetings will help keep it on the front burner for them.

Principle Three: High Utilization Targets Encourage High Utilization

Don't be afraid to aim high in setting targets for utilization. If your initial utilization goals are low, you can rest assured that your organization's utilization level will be low. If your initial goals are high, end-users may be encouraged to meet them.

Of course, modest goals are safer than grand targets, but is a safe success better than a risky failure? Answering that question is a matter of internal politics but even if the leadership won't support a 100 percent utilization goal, complete utilization should at least be viewed as a plausible long-term goal.

No matter what utilization goal you finally establish, be sure that it is clearly defined and easily understood by everyone involved in the implementation. When President John F. Kennedy pledged to put a man on the moon, it was a goal that would stretch the resources and expertise of NASA to the breaking point. But no one in the Houston control room complained that the goal was intangible or difficult to understand.

Principle Four: Experience is the Best Teacher

An old proverb advises us to "learn from others' mistakes (because) life is too short to make them all yourself." One simple way to learn from the EHR experiences of other health care organizations is to create a steering committee whose membership draws from many different fields and/or departments across your organization. Each steering committee member will bring with them valuable knowledge garnered from other technology projects (ideally, EHR projects).

Another highly recommended practice is to conduct site visits of organizations that have already deployed an EHR. On these visits, which typically take place during the sales process or very early in the implementation process, keep an eye out for utilization clues such as the number of physicians using the EHR, the organization's patient mix, specialties, and payers. Such experience can help prepare staff for advanced training, thus making the training more effective.

Principle Five: Theories are only as Good as Their Results

While you're looking around for industry examples to learn from, remember that what works for one organization may not work for another. If you find a good idea that seems to work in another setting, give it a shot. But be ready to abandon it if it doesn't work, or if changing conditions affect its early success. Remember, flexibility is a virtue. When your initial theory or strategy appears to be slowing, don't be afraid to change horses mid-stream. The strategy that got you to 50-percent utilization might not have the legs to get you to 100 percent.

> **VITALS**
>
> **If required skills are weak in the organization, don't let that impact your utilization goals. Get training and/or seek consulting assistance from an expert in the defined target areas.**

The theory of diminishing returns will eventually come into play with any strategy. Take a not-so-hypothetical example. Let's say an organization adopts an initial implementation strategy of bringing every physician up on the EHR at one time. The strategy works brilliantly for the first two months and the numbers indicate the organization will soon reach full utilization. But after three months the numbers begin to dive, then nosedive. Recognizing that changing circumstances were undermining their initial utilization strategy, the organization responded by deploying additional EHR modules, with a strong focus on one-to-one training and physician support. The new approach turned out to have more lasting power and within a few months the organization had achieved its utilization goals.

Principle Six: Utilization Promotion Only Works If You Work It

Deploying an EHR is a highly complex endeavor that can take years to complete. After several months or a year you might begin to wonder what happened to those EHR pieces that were deployed with a target utilization rate of 50 percent. As new pieces of the EHR were implemented, did anyone revisit those goals and perhaps raise the target rate? Careful consideration of your own deployment must include continuous updating and reevaluation of utilization goals and targets. For instance, as more physicians begin to use more EHR modules, they'll reveal greater efficiencies and better utilization strategies—and this growing body of information will make it easier to quickly improve utilization. And yet, none of these efficiencies or strategies will be realized unless you are constantly assessing and refining.

Principle Seven: Financial Incentives Aren't Magic Bullets

It's important to balance the carrot and the stick. Even though some organizations have been able to effectively leverage financial incentives to increase utilization, incentives are by no means the only sure-fire way to achieve success. In fact, the last thing you need is a political battle over employee contracts dividing physicians and management. Such divisiveness could jeopardize the entire project, which requires sound teamwork and a shared commitment to succeed. Bear in mind, too, that some physicians are motivated more by achievement, individual empowerment, or status than financial gain, so from the organization's perspective it's imperative that the physician's group be regarded both as a group and as a combination of individuals with differing ambitions and needs. Best practice organizations are able to direct and steer the energy of their individuals toward the completion of objectives defined by the organization.

As you can see from these seven principles, there are no shortcuts to high utilization. It's going to be a long, hard road. Still, by sticking to these principles you'll be halfway to your destination. The next step is to use the principles to build a utilization management program that's based on best practices from successful EHR implementations.

Building a Program for Utilization Management

"When your only tool is a hammer, every problem looks like a nail."

A strong utilization management plan has its roots in the very beginning of the implementation—the EHR shopping spree. A core buying requirement for the EHR should be that the solution promotes general usage. Ask prospective vendors to produce evidence that their solutions are compatible with a strong utilization program based on defined interventions, not simply luck. By adhering to this strategy, you are in a sense buying utilization and avoiding the later costs associated with poor utilization.

After incorporating utilization principles into the purchasing process, the next step in laying the foundation for a utilization management plan is to convene a working group on utilization. Ideally, the team should include the Executive Sponsor, the Project Manager, and the Physician Sponsor. With help from this group, you can build a plan that's compatible with your EHR solution and all segments of the organization, from management down to the end-users. A guiding principle for the working group should be inclusiveness of all points of view in the decision-making process. To support this principle as the working group moves forward, it should avoid making organizational-level decisions unless a quorum is present.

In formulating the utilization management plan, think first of strategies that will appeal to your customer base, the physicians. What's important to them? For example, when trying to drive physician adoption, it's a good idea to begin by implementing an activity that physicians are already familiar with, such as dictation (assuming your EHR allows you to deploy modules one at a time, not all at once). Because the EHR will enable faster, easier dictation, providers will quickly become comfortable with the application and the use of any new devices that may go along with the system, such as PDAs or Tablet PCs. And the high adoption rate of a dictation module can demonstrate success early on and ease the adoption of later modules.

Strategies from the Real World

Now that we've laid the foundation for a utilization management program, let's examine some real-world utilization strategies. The following examples from actual EHR implementations offer a glimpse into what has already been attempted but they are by no means exhaustive. There are many different ways to deploy a strategy and in the end every organization has a way of making a strategy uniquely theirs. So be critical in examining these strategies. Ask yourself, what would you do differently? Can you identify strategies that would work in your organization or, perhaps more important, strategies that would fail? Thinking critically will help you create a customized plan designed specifically for your organization.

Organization Type: Surgical group with divisions (40+ Physicians)

1. Identify and appoint Physician Sponsors for each specialty division. (A primary Physician Sponsor leads these division sponsors, but it's important to have a point of contact for each division)

2. Roll out deployment plan, including responsibilities for Physician Sponsors

3. Go "live" with the EHR in the smallest division first (based on the number of physicians)

4. Physician Sponsor for the division acts as support and/or peer mentor, as well as the first point of contact

5. Incrementally, based on their size (smallest to largest), divisions continue to go live

6. Previous divisions help encourage utilization in later divisions by:

   a) Sharing their successes and failures

   b) Demonstrating that it was a fairly painless process

   c) Communicating what worked

   d) Discussing pitfalls

7. Deployment team notes successes and pitfalls and adjusts strategy accordingly as the roll-out continues

8. Build experience and confidence incrementally as rollouts continue with the EHR

Organization Type: Orthopedic Group (20+ Physicians)

1. Identify and appoint a Physician Sponsor for the entire group

2. Plan limited rollout

3. Initially, only early adopters go live with the EHR

4. Other physicians go live in groups of two or three at a time, which allows for:

   a) More individualized support as doctors begin to use the EHR

   b) Improved physician comfort levels with the technology

   c) Some hand-holding of resistant doctors

Note: Strong, one-on-one support at the time of the go live made this deployment strategy and EHR adoption successful.

Organization Type: Multi-Specialty Group (50+ Physicians)

1. Clearly define ROI goals for the EHR (taking care to include non-monetary goals that will appeal directly to physicians, such as ease of access to the patient chart and work time-savings)

2. Perform preliminary measurements and cost analyses

3. Go live with selected doctors

4. Perform post-implementation measurement

5. Share ROI advantages with other physicians in the practice.

6. Other physicians are motivated by a compelling ROI success story

Further Methods for Driving Physician Utilization

As these examples indicate, a utilization management plan doesn't have to be overly complex to be effective; it just has to fit the organization. A case in point: The final example above is from a large multi-specialty physician practice. The organization's strategy for driving physician utilization was almost completely driven by return on investment metrics, which allowed the project team to clearly see numerical measurements of utilization as the implementation progressed. By extracting accurate measures from early rollouts to physicians, management was able to demonstrate to the practice's other physicians the ROI and financial benefits from active use of the EHR. The organization's strategy worked primarily because the practice's management team knew their physicians and recognized that an emphasis on ROI would get their attention and win their support for the implementation.

Another good way to drive physician utilization is to configure the EHR to make it easy for physicians to access the tools they use most often throughout the day. Popular tools that can be pre-loaded into an EHR include favorites lists for commonly prescribed medicines, problems, and charge codes. This approach to driving utilization focuses on making it easier for physicians to do their jobs more quickly, which has the added benefit of improving patient care.

Still another way to drive utilization is to communicate the qualitative and quantitative benefits of utilization of the EHR. Both types of benefits appeal to physicians' interest in providing high quality care while also improving the quality of their work lives.

Common qualitative benefits of the EHR include:

- Enabling physicians to spend more time in the exam room, and to complete "paperwork" at home in the evenings via Web portal access to charts.
- Increased patient safety. Several recent studies indicate the frequency of medical errors can be significantly reduced through the use of EHR tools such as e-prescribing, automatic drug-interaction checking, and clinical guidelines alerts.

Common quantitative benefits include:

- Savings in operating costs from new process efficiencies
- Generation of new revenues from proper E/M coding, which can prevent down coding and reduces the incidence of denials of claims.
- Timesavings due to instant access to patient charts.

Extracting Metrics to Drive Utilization

Because an EHR lets you extract meaningful usage data infinitely more quickly than with paper records, you can measure the statistical utilization of the new system quite easily. For instance, you could identify utilization trends across different products, or by specialty. And you can identify individuals who over-use or under-use the EHR.

To take advantage of the EHR's metrics' extraction capabilities, first define utilization progress measures that are important to your clinic and compare these measures to the desired outcomes. This comparison will help to maximize your investment in the EHR by revealing areas in need of improvement, as well as successful strategies that can be applied to other areas. Don't forget to tell the users what you're going to be measuring. Good communication on your part helps them to know what to expect.

Now that you've discovered how gathering statistics can aid utilization management, you need to keep doing it! This isn't a one-time shot. Use your new reports every week to monitor progress and keep an eye on individuals and groups. You may *think* that the users are all entering their prescriptions, charges, and orders into the system, but the statistical data will tell you the whole story. Don't let perceptions fool you. Just because everyone gives the appearance of using the EHR doesn't mean that they're *really* using it. Let the data speak for itself and then share it with your organization.

Measuring Utilization Success

Measuring the success (or failure) of your utilization program is similar to measuring return on investment from the EHR, a topic we covered in Chapter Five. It involves gathering current metrics and comparing them to a pre-EHR baseline. Rather than comparing dollars and cents, however, or looking for signs

VITALS: PHYSICIANS APPRECIATE BENEFITS

There's no better way to convince physicians to adopt the EHR than by showing them its physician-centric benefits:

- Elimination of "down-coding," the act of choosing less restrictive and lower compensated reimbursement codes for ambulatory charges.
- Better access to the patient's chart as there is no longer a need to pull the chart and no more "missing" charts. The chart is always available to view through the EHR from the office or from home, even when another doctor or nurse is viewing it.
- Documents become part of the chart faster. It has been shown that scanning and electronically filing a document is more efficient than manually filing.
- Faster return for transcribed dictations either through direct input via dictation markers or through automated transcription processes.
- Reduction in the exposure to medical liability as the EHR offers the ability to provide high levels of documentation, through the use of standardized clinical terminology such as the content found in the MEDCIN database, and auditing.

of improvements in quality, you'll be testing whether physicians are using the new system as expected.

Begin by establishing baseline reference points before the implementation. You'll need to measure the routine, paper-based clinical tasks that you expect to be most powerfully affected by the EHR, such as the number of prescriptions written, or the number of transcriptions. Which measurements you take will depend on your organizational goals and objectives, outlined in the Project Scope document (see Chapter Six). If one of the organization's goals is to get 95 percent of physicians using the EHR within one year of implementation, then you might want to collect data on the number and percentage of physicians using the EHR, or how many of the system's modules they're using. Success, or lack of it, will again be measured according to the goals and objectives outlined in the scope document.

The following is a sample of metrics that can be collected from a database-based EHR system. These samples are broken down into three different levels according to the database reporting structure of a typical EHR product.

Sample EHR Metrics

Account Level (data pertinent to the overall system)

- Number of active users
- Number of documents scanned into the system

Provider Level (data pertinent to the tasks and activities of physicians and other providers in the system), for each individual provider:

- Number of Arrived Patients
- Number of Prescriptions authorized through the EHR
- Number of charges billed
- Number of dictations created
- Number of minutes dictated
- Number of orders authorized
- Number of scanned documents viewed
- Number of forms created
- Number of unstructured notes created

- Number of unstructured notes signed
- Number of structured notes created
- Number of structured notes signed
- Number of new results in the system

User Level—data pertinent to the tasks and activities of Users in the system

- Number of transcriptions entered into the system

Utilization Reports

The following figures illustrate what utilization reports might look like based on system and user information in the EHR system. In fact, these mock reports are based on utilization reports extracted from an EHR system in use in today's market. From the report in Figure 1 we can easily view data compiled across the entire organization for a number of different data categories related to both module usage and system usage. The data in this report gives analysts an overview of utilization numbers for the entire organization.

In Figure 2, we can view detailed data separated out by the individual physician. These types of metrics make it easy to compare and contrast EHR usage by physicians, as well as examine individual usage trends and characteristics. The information can be used to answer important questions about system utilization. Do users need additional training? What do we need to do to bring the numbers up? If Dr. X has viewed 1,000 scanned images whereas Dr. Y has only viewed 100, how can Dr. X's EHR workflow help others to better utilize the information in the system?

Access to such useful utilization data helps facilitate new strategies and improvements to old strategies. It's also helpful in uncovering trouble spots and utilization challenges. For instance, if the utilization numbers on processed prescriptions are still low after implementing a prescription module, there are three possible causes: 1) users need more training; 2) the system and workflow may need additional configuration; or 3) users still have access to their old methods and have reverted to using them.

Organization Data Report

	# of Clinical Users	# of Licensed Providers	# of Arrived Patients	# of RXs	# of Dictations	Dictation Minutes	# of Signed Documents	# of Scanned Documents	# of Forms Created	# of Documents Created	# of Charges	# of Orders	# of Signed Notes	# of Results
Region: East														
XYZ Clinic	132	92	9599	1986	3	1	3073	4839	0	7089	0	5505	1689	3659
East Region Total	132	92	9599	1986	3	1	3073	4839	0	7089	0	5505	1689	3659

Diagram 1. A bird's eye view of the organization's EHR usage

Data By Provider

XYZ Clinic

Date Range: 9/1/2004 - 12/1/2004

Specialty: All Specialties
Provider: All Providers

	# of Arrived Patients	# of RXs	# of Dictations	Dictation Minutes	# of Documents Created	# of Documents Signed	# of Forms Created	# of Scanned Documents Viewed	# of Notes Created	# of Notes Signed	# of Charges	# of Orders	# of Results
W	905	465	0	0	1089	941	0	0	221	117	0	0	0
P	1001	524	52	153	654	1230	0	789	233	201	454	132	57

Diagram 2. Utilization numbers for individual providers

In summary, you can help to ensure the long-term success of the EHR implementation by revisiting utilization levels on a regular basis. Moving from inception to full deployment, enforce the gradual inclusion of utilization as expected behavior through the governance and administrative mechanisms of the practice. Leverage existing policies and, when possible, incorporate usage of the EHR into these policies. Use metrics to determine what is working and where the challenges lie, and then keep those numbers going up. Relate you successes and milestones to the organization. Give closure to implementation sections and phases. Use these calm points in the deployment to review the current state of things, pick up those users who may have been left behind, and fine-tune your utilization management plan.

Overcoming Challenges to Utilization

The Chinese character for "challenge" also means "opportunity." On your way to achieving your utilization goals, you'll face plenty of challenges. In responding to them, try to uncover the opportunities for constructive change that they represent. Another way of saying the same thing is that every failure is a signpost to success. For instance, the primary reason why efforts to boost physician utilization fail is that adoption is not mandated, and creating a sense of project ownership by the physicians is not cultivated by the organization. In our experience, this is a big mistake. The changeover from paper to electronic records is such a major undertaking that, if it is not mandatory or if doctors do not feel a strong connection and commitment to the project's success, they're likely to offer resistance.

To make utilization mandatory, first set plausible deadlines for transferring clinical and administrative processes to the EHR. At Affinity Health Group, management mandated that all new patient information be entered into the EHR on the day it went live. Affinity simply refused to let physicians create any new paper records. Within a matter of months, physicians no longer wanted to access the old, paper chart because it was hopelessly out-of-date.

Of course, there are many other challenges to implementing and utilizing an EHR. Let's take a closer look at the real challenges you'll face.

Playbook on How to Fail with an EHR Deployment

What does a failed deployment have to do with your utilization management plan? By examining others' failures, you can learn how to succeed. The following data was compiled from twenty EHR deployments by several vendors between 2002 and 2004. As Figure 3 illustrates, four of the implementations were considered failures; four were deemed complete successes; and twelve resulted in some level of success.

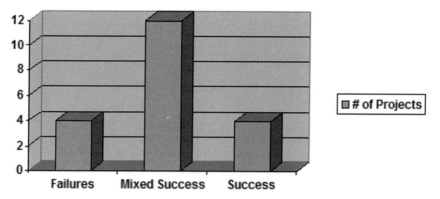

Results from twenty EHR implementations, 2002-2004

Not surprisingly, all the failures shared common traits. But some of these common traits were quite surprising. As you read through the list of actual implementation results below, take a moment to ponder the scenarios. Confronted by a similar situation, would you be able to avoid pitfalls? And would you be willing to listen to difficult advice, even if it meant changing your strategy?

Common Reasons Why EHR Deployments Fail:

- The executive team insisted upon an all-at-once implementation (all of their physicians went live with the EHR simultaneously) and there was minimal internal leadership to get the physicians involved in training or to help with design and setup of the system. The executive leadership determined goals and priorities without physician involvement.

- The organization lacked strong physician and user support for change, although they were enthusiastic about the novelty of the technology.

- The implementation timeline was too short and unaligned with the goals of the deployment.

- There was no internal steering committee.

- The project team's relationship to providers was that of outsiders.

- Physicians never played an active role in system design or simulation testing.

- No specific measurable goals were defined for ROI.

- No pre-live or post-live measurements were taken.

- End users were not aware of goals and ROI results were not communicated regularly to end-users after go-live.

- Physicians' use of the EHR was optional and not incentivized.

- Project team members rarely if ever returned communications to the EHR vendor.

- Deployments were all single-phase (modules were not phased in a few at a time).

- The EHR rollout took less than six months.

Many of these common traits speak for themselves, but the central conclusion confirms one of the main theses of this book—to develop a successful EHR project, you must involve the physicians. (One side note: Surprisingly, no one listed funding or budget constraints as a cause of failure, even though industry studies show these are two of the biggest problems confronting implementations).

Playbook on How to Succeed with an EHR Deployment

Now that we've seen what *doesn't* work, let's discuss what it takes to succeed. The following list was compiled from the EHR projects deemed to be complete successes.

VITALS: WHAT IF ORGANIZATIONAL RESOLVE TO UTILIZATION MANAGEMENT WEAKENS?

Revisit and rededicate your organization to required outcomes. Identify causes for decline and create solutions. Evaluate your processes, key factors, and key actors for possible changes.

Common Reasons Why EHR Deployments Succeed:

- The EHR was deployed in multiple phases, not all at once.
- The EHR rollout took between six and twelve months.
- The deployment timeframe was realistic in relation to resources.
- The Physician Sponsor had prior EHR experience.
- Half of the projects had internal steering committees.
- The project team's relationship to physicians and end-users was classified as either "insiders/very close" or "outsiders, but frequent interaction."
- Pre-live and post-live measurements were taken.
- End-users were made aware of goals before going live with the EHR.
- Physicians and end-users were informed of any new, post-live process changes early and often.
- High levels of communication were maintained between the vendor and the customer.
- Physicians were motivated to utilize the EHR either by mandating usage or through financial incentives.

Although putting all of these elements in place does not guarantee project success, these characteristics are the essential ingredients of a healthy EHR implementation. Many of the characteristics also support a successful utilization program (e.g., an experienced Physician Sponsor, emphasis on metrics, and especially, physician motivators).

Minimizing Perceived Roadblocks

Perceived roadblocks are really nothing more (or less) than negative feelings—powerful emotional responses to the EHR. Many people find that a new task or duty, such as adopting an EHR, can elicit fear, distrust, dread, trepidation, or doubt. As we mentioned in Chapter Nine, those plagued by these negative feelings can easily become unconscious saboteurs of the project and its utilization. If their emotions cause them to spread hearsay, rumor, idle speculation, and suspicion about the project, then they have become the harbingers of failure.

Why would anyone want to sabotage the EHR? Typically, they fear the new system will make them look foolish or incompetent in front of their colleagues, or patients. Let's face it—change isn't easy. When you attempt something new (especially if it's a complicated undertaking like an EHR), you assume that it will take some time before you become proficient and quite a long time before you become an expert.

Given the high potential for emotional difficulties during an EHR implementation, it's important to know your organization's mental health status. As we discussed in Chapter Nine, to understand organizational behavior, you need to understand employee commitment, psychological ownership, perceived control, leadership traits, and overall corporate culture, among other things. Having a corporate culture that embraces technological change will certainly help in achieving high levels of utilization with an EHR. But if your organization's tolerance for technological change is low, you can still succeed. You just have to recognize the situation and take it into consideration when planning your implementation and utilization program.

A good plan for preventing and circumventing perceived roadblocks focuses on communication and education. A direct approach is best. Clinical phobias are often treated by a gradual process of exposure to the object of the fear. Similarly, you can expose those with a low tolerance for technological change to the EHR in a safe environment, accompanied by their peers. Help them to feel comfortable with the technology and the workflow, to learn about the product and its use. Provide education and consultation, and access to other sites internally and externally where the same EHR product is deployed. And encourage users to participate in vendor and product-specific user groups.

Perceived roadblocks can impede progress just as surely as the real ones. Don't let fear and emotion detract from the positive reality of high utilization. The best strategy is to learn from the roadblocks you encounter and use what you learn to improve the utilization program.

Building the Bridge

Throughout this chapter, we've used and reused the theme of "definition, identification, communication, and inclusion." They are the foundation of a strong utilization plan. Learn from others whenever possible and make utilization a priority that receives continuous evaluation, scrutiny, and improvement. Analysis and application of pertinent metrics should be employed whenever possible to drive utilization. Recognize the driving forces and persuasions that affect physician adoption and make careful consideration of your own organization's nature and culture.

In the end, utilization management is an all-the-time concern that must be based on sharp observation of reality and intelligent analysis, not hopes and wishes. Now that you've witnessed the archetypes of utilization management it's time to go out and build your own utilization suspension bridge. Let your plan lead your organization from implementation dreams to the reality of goals realized.

The Recap

- Success centers on the Physicians. Physician inclusion, and an EHR geared to their needs, will help ensure high utilization.
- Utilization management is an all-the-time concern of the leadership team. It must be kept on the agenda or utilization potential will not be attained.
- Learn from a variety of experiences, yours and others. Investigate others' failures, as well as successes and incorporate the lessons into your plan.
- Assess and refine utilization promotion programs. Revisit your utilization management strategy and make adjustments.
- Utilizing the EHR will expand your physicians' tool set. Leverage new capabilities.
- Use metrics to promote utilization levels. Analysis of "hard" data extracted from the EHR will assist in targeting areas of success and challenge.
- Perceived roadblocks can impede progress just as surely as the real ones. Don't let fear and emotion detract from the positive reality of high utilization.

If You Have The Time

- Cost-Justifying Electronic Medical Records. Kevin Renner. Healthcare Financial Management (1996).

- The Economic Effect of Implementing and EHR in an Outpatient Clinical Setting. S. Barlow, J. Johnson, and J. Steck. Journal of Healthcare Information Management (Winter 2004).

- A Cost-Benefit Analysis of Electronic Medical Records in Primary Care. S.J. Wang, B. Middleton and others. American Journal of Medicine (April 2003).

- The end of autonomy? Reflections on the Post-professional Physician. Stephen J. O'Connor, and Joyce A. Lanning. Health Care Management Review (Winter 1992).

Sample Resource Responsibilities and Qualifications

Base-Level Staffing Table

Application System Administrator

Responsibilities	Qualifications and Skills
Support Responsibilities: • Overall responsibility for maintaining the EHR configuration on a day-to-day basis, for small-scale rollout/new users and for application upgrades • Coordinate client resources, as needed, for application upgrades and other system projects that occur during steady-state operations of the Advance phase. • Escalation path for front-line end-user support resources • Primary contact for EHR vendor's support services • If a separate resource from implementation team, assist building system configuration during implementation	• 1+ years of clinical experience • 1+ years at customer site • Ability to effectively communicate with clinicians • Strong analytical skills • Excellent organization skills • Technical aptitude • High-level understanding of EHR technical environment • Trained on use and administration of all applicable EHR functionality

Business/Ancillary Systems Management

Responsibilities	Qualifications and Skills
• Generates enthusiasm for software • Lead workflow redesign and implementation rollout efforts within department • Become thoroughly familiar with the product features/capabilities and future-state workflows • Promote project goals/strategy to department to enhance adoption by physicians and staff • Provide the clinical/business expertise for set up decisions • Review current policies/procedures and update accordingly for new post-live workflows • Review internal training curriculum and materials • Develop clinical/business workflow testing scenarios and perform testing	• 2+ years industry experience • 1+ years experience at customer site • Extensive knowledge of clinical workflows • Decision making capabilities with empowerment for assigned areas • Strong Analytical/Problem Solving skills • Change Management skills

Client Device Support

Responsibilities	Qualifications and Skills
Implementation/support responsibilities: • Ensure all client devices (PCs, PDAs, etc) are supported • Ensure all client devices are maintained to the requirements of the EHR solution • Provide client device support to end-users	• 1+ years field experience • 1+ years at customer site • Decision making skills • Technical skills • Knowledge of customer/server/networks and PC's • Excellent communication and organizational skills

Responsibilities	Qualifications and Skills
• Function as change agents during the implementation within their clinic/location • Communicate business and functional needs during the implementation process • Champion the migration to our solutions and ensure their respective departments and functional areas are prepared to utilize the solutions. • Within their domain of expertise and working side by side with core project team members: ✓ Attend training sessions ✓ Actively communicate design requirements and participate in design sessions. ✓ Ensure Design is validated with key stakeholders from their areas ✓ Execute the system "Build" Activities for their respective area of expertise/ assignment and ensure the build complies with all design elements and quality measures ✓ Work closely with and or execute Testing and Training functions to ensure all necessary components and plans are developed, executed and measured for quality and completeness ✓ Participate in Simulation Activities ✓ Assist with the development and execution of Go-live preparation and tasks.	• Respected by peers • Flexible and accepting of evolving new processes and change • Demonstrated understanding of business environment • Analytical skills • Understanding of software and technology and help peers with translation and transition • Ability to convince peers that the value is worth the effort, focusing on quality of care • "Thick Skin" and willing to stay the course • Team should represent all user roles being implemented (such as physicians, nurses, front desk, lab, business office)

Clinical Advisory Board

Responsibilities	Qualifications and Skills
If separated from the EHR Steering Committee: • Lead change with peers and make timely clinical design decisions • Participate in creation of system configuration and content loading strategies, as required • Responsible for sign-off on clinical design and configuration	• Influential in the physician and/or clinical management community • Comfortable with technology, not necessarily an expert • Understand cross-organizational objectives and can represent department or specialty requirements

EHR Steering Committee

Responsibilities	Qualifications and Skills
• Responsible for ensuring organizational enablers are in place and functioning • Lead change and make timely decisions • Makes cross organizational decisions and resolves conflicting needs/ issues • Escalation point for key project governance decisions • Escalation point for key project and system design and configuration decisions • Responsible for all final decisions and acceptance of the project's product.	• Typically chaired by the Executive Sponsor • Key clinical, operational and implementation task force leads • Representation should minimally include Physician leadership, Clinic management and the management leaders of the operational departments affected by the EHR implementation (business office, compliance, medical records, information systems, etc.)

End-user Application Support and/or Help-desk

Responsibilities	Qualifications and Skills
Support Responsibilities: • Primary phone and/or on-site application support for end-users • Coordinate escalation with system administrator, IS lead and Interface analyst	• 1+ year of industry experience • Ability to effectively communicate with clinicians • Strong analytical skills • Strong technical aptitude • Trained and certified on use of all applicable EHR functionality

Executive Sponsor

Responsibilities	Qualifications and Skills
• Ensures project goals align with organizational goals • Responsible for organizational readiness and ensuring enablers are functioning as planned • Provides overall direction for project • Responsible for presenting final acceptance and project approval to the sponsor(s)	• Has direct decision-making authority for the majority of issues the project manager may need to escalate • Excellent communication and organizational skills • Excellent team facilitation skills • Comfortable with technology, not necessarily an expert

Integration and Conversion Analyst

Responsibilities	Qualifications and Skills
• Analyze/Communicate the practice management system/3rd-Party System integration requirements • Review interface specifications • Provide the analytical expertise for set up decisions • Gather and write iterative interface test scenarios • Participate in integration testing and issue resolution • Assist Project Manager in system rollout planning from an integration perspective • Manage dictionary maintenance between the EHR solution and other systems **Implementation/support responsibilities:** • Monitor all interfaces and connectivity • Monitor/resolve interface error logs • Primary contact for interface alerts	• 2+ years industry experience • 1+ years at the customer site • Excellent communication and organizational skills • Analytical skills • Technical aptitude

IS Lead

Responsibilities	Qualifications and Skills
Implementation/support responsibilities: • Oversee all technical aspects of the installation and support • Act as primary customer contact for your EHR vendor Technical Resources • Drive technical implementation and on-going support to meet success criteria and goals • Act as liaison between your EHR vendor and third-party vendors	• 3-5 years field experience • 1+ years at customer site • 2+ years Microsoft-based server/networking administration experience • Decision making skills • Technical skills • Knowledge of servers, networks and PC's • Excellent communication skills

Network Administrator

Responsibilities	Qualifications and Skills
Implementation/support responsibilities: • Ensure that LAN/WAN meets requirements, is operational and supported • RF Network Implementation and Support, when applicable • Maintain environment security • Work with your EHR vendor Network team to provide and support remote connectivity	• 3-5 years field experience • 1+ years at customer site • 2+ years Microsoft-centric network administration experience • Decision making skills • Technical skills • Knowledge of customer/server/networks and PC's • Excellent communication and organizational skills

Physician Sponsor

Responsibilities	Qualifications and Skills
• Generates enthusiasm for software • Provides guidance and makes decisions regarding the business and clinical needs • Reviews software functionality regularly • Sits on the EHR Steering Committee	• Influential in the physician community • Excellent communication and organizational skills • Comfortable with technology, not necessarily an expert

Project Manager

Responsibilities	Qualifications and Skills
Separate project managers may be utilized for initial implementation and rollout depending on the proposed deployment strategy and number of physicians. • Oversee and coordinate all aspects of the implementation project and it's deliverables – ensuring a high quality implementation • Act as primary customer contact for your EHR vendor • Facilitate decision making within the organization • Drive implementation project to meet success criteria and goals • Facilitates issue management and resolution • Ensure communication across departmental project teams and end users • Attend project team training and be thoroughly familiar with the product features/capabilities and future-state workflows	• 3 – 5 years project management experience • 1+ years experience at customer site • Proven decision maker • Demonstrated leadership and motivation skills • Excellent communication and organizational skills • Analytical skills • Technical aptitude • Can asses risk and develop corrective action plans • Change Management skills

Server & Database Administrator

Responsibilities	Qualifications and Skills
Implementation/support responsibilities: • Assist with initial setup of server • Work with Technical representative to ensure proper system backups meet or exceed your EHR vendor's recommended strategy • Ensure that system protection software is up to date • Perform daily system maintenance (Monitoring, backups, etc.)	• 3-5 years field experience • 1+ years at customer site • 2+ years programming experience • Decision making skills • Technical skills • Knowledge of customer/server/networks and PC's • Excellent communication and organizational skills

Training Coordinator and Trainers

Responsibilities	Qualifications and Skills
• Assesses end-user training needs and resources • Develops training approach and plan • Learns products and associated processes • Participates in Design and Build sessions • Works with department managers to review policies and to develop new work-flows • Develops internal training curriculum and materials • Coordinates training resources • Provides on-going end-user and new employee training • Provide on-site support during initial go-live on new functionality	• 1-3 years training experience • 1+ years experience at customer site • Demonstrated use of training methods • Excellent communication and organizational skills • Good PC skills • Demonstrated understanding of clinical workflows

CLINIC LEADERSHIP

Role	Base-level Staffing	Allocation	Staffing Variations
Physician Champion	1	10% (During local implementation)	Increase for each specialty and/or clinic.
Clinical Champions	2-4	10-20 % (During local implementation)	Increase for each specialty and/or clinic.
Operational Champions	1-3	10-20 % (During local implementation)	Increase for each specialty resident at each clinic.

Role	Base-level Staffing	Allocation	Staffing Variations
Project Manager	1	100 %	A second PM may be added for simultaneous new implementations with phased rollout, or two project coordinators (implementation and rollout) can be placed under the guidance of a single Project Manager.
Clinical and operational specialists	1 - 3	80-100%	Expand as needed to provide a strong base of cross-organizational expertise. Temporary resources may be added to this group to facilitate data entry during system configuration.
Business/Ancillary Systems' Management	1 - 2	20 – 40 % System design and configuration	Expand as needed to adequately cover clinical and business operations expertise. This role typically includes participation from billing, laboratory, radiology, pharmacy managers, etc, as applicable.
Training Coordinator/trainer	1	20-50 % System design and configuration 100 % Live and Post-live	Variation will occur dependent on the rollout strategy, however the following guidelines can be used as an estimation: 1 per 25 providers 1 per 50 end-users Note: It is recommended to outsource supplemental training resources to cover periods of peak implementation and rollout.
Integration and conversion analyst(s)	1 – 2	50 – 80% System design and configuration	Resource allocation is dependent on the number of interfaces and/or conversions with third-party systems.
IS lead	1	50%	

Role	Base-level Staffing	Allocation	Staffing Variations
Executive Sponsor	1	20 %	
Physician Sponsor(s)	1	20 – 30 %	2 – 3 per 100 providers
EHR Steering Committee	TBD	5 – 10 %	Based on your leadership structure. Should include representation from appropriate operational leaders impacted by the EHR. Minimum recommendation is a twice-monthly meeting, including executive and Physician Sponsors, and the Project Manager. (This may become a monthly meeting in later phases of implementation).
Clinical Advisory Board	TBD	5 – 10%	Representative physician and clinical management involvement from each department or specialty.

IS Support Team

Role	Base-level Staffing	Allocation	Staffing Variations
Practice Management / Third-Party System Analysts	1-3	10 – 20%	Varies based on the EHR functionality and systems being integrated. Representation primarily for considerations with patient access, billing, and ancillary systems.
Network Administrator	1	10 %	Variation is based on the level of compliance with the EHR network specifications.
Server/Database Administrator	1	20 %	
Client device support	1	100 %	1 per 300 devices
Application System Administrator	1	50 – 100%	The Project Manager or trainer may transition into this role.
End-user application support and/or help-desk	1	100 %	1 per 200 end-users (that have been live more than 3 months). Additional support required during initial rollout weeks.

APPENDIX TWO

ROI Chart

ROI Measures

The following list of ROI Measurables can be used to provide a framework of items available for EHR ROI analysis. This list is by no means meant to be an exhaustive representation of all measurable items, but merely a guideline. The list is separated into 3 areas concerning the chart, coding, and transcription. Items in italics represent where a calculated measure resulting from the combination of corresponding measurements could be made.

CHART ASSOCIATED SAVINGS

RN Time for Chart Responsibilities (Reallocation of Time)

	FTEs (Total Number of Nurses, NPs, PAs)
	% of RN Time Spent on Chart Responsibilities
	FTEs Expense (Indirect Chart Responsibilites)
	Reduction in Chart Pulls and Other Activities (%)
	Savings in RN Time Due to Reduction in Chart Pulls

Staff Time in Pulling Charts

	Number of Chart Pulls for Scheduled Patients (daily)
	Number of Chart Pulls for Ad hoc requests(daily)
	Total Chart Pulls (daily)
	Total Chart Pulls (annually)
	Cost per Chart Pull
	Annual Cost for Chart Pulls
	Reduction in Chart Pulls (%)
	Projected Decrease in Staffing Due to Effiencies
	Decrease in Staff Required for Pulling, Filing and Maintaining Charts

Development of New Charts

	Number of New Charts Developed (annually)
	Cost per Chart Developed
	Cost for Developing New Charts (annual)
	Eliminate the Need to Develop Charts for New Patients

Supply Costs

	Superbills
	Rx pads
	Folders
	Courier Costs
	Labels
	Subtotal
	Estimated Reduction
	Reduction in Supply Expenses

CODING

	% of visits downcoded
	Average loss/pt.
	Average loss/day
	Annual Improvement - Potential
	Estimated utilization
	Increase in Coding Levels and Revenue Due to Improved Documentation

TRANSCRIPTION

	Annual Dictation Expenses
	Estimated Reduction
	Reduction in Transcription Expenses

APPENDIX THREE

Sample Communication Plan

[Project Name] Communication Plan						
What	**To Whom**	**When**	**Who**	**How**	**Where**	**Comments**
Initial Communication	Clinic Management and physicians	After contract..	Executive Champion	Established Newsletter, flyer, something tangible	Physical inboxes, break rooms, lounges and high traffic areas	Establish frequency of communication. Offer opportunity for Q&A, open forums, etc.
	All Clinic Staff	After Kick-off..	Executive Champion/Physician Champion	Established Newsletter, flyer, something tangible	Physical inboxes, break rooms, lounges and high traffic areas	
Key area Information Sessions						
Regional/Local Support Sessions						
Feedback opportunity						Round trip with every person to discuss design, get individual feedback and answer questions.
						Mechanism to provide comments and suggestions about material, design and new ideas.
Corporate Information Sessions						Create awareness through out business unit on challenges being addressed, modifications and overall terminology
Cycle will repeat when new components or iterations of the design are rolled out internally.						

Resource Assignment Matrix

Resource Assignment Matrix
(Key: O = Owner; C = Contributor; A = Acceptance; R = Reviewer)

(Insert Client Name)   (Insert Vendor Name)

Deliverable	Project Manager	Applications Analyst	Interface Analyst	Trainer	Technical Manager	Technical Team	Help Desk Manager / System Administrator	End-User Change / Rollout Manager	Physician Champions / Clinical Provider SMEs	Executive Sponsor	Steering Committee	Project Manager	Implementation Consultant
Introduction													
Project Intro Call	A / C											O	C
Technical Intro Call	C				A / C							C	
Interface Intro Call	C		A / C									C	
Organizational Prep													
Document Project Goals, Success Criteria, ROI metrics & measurement process	O	C	C	C	C		C	C	C	C	A	R	
Organizational Data Gathering	O	C	C	C	C			C		C	C		
Hardware Prep													
Data Center Preparation	R				O	C							
Hardware Installation	R				O	C							
Planning for End-User Training													
End-User Training Plan	R				O			C		A		R	R
Trainer Dress Rehearsal	A	R			O							R	R
System Testing													
Test Environment Testing	O	C	C	C	C								R
End-User Simulation (in TEST)	O	C		C					A			R	R
Live Environment Testing	O	C	C	C	C								R
End-User Acceptance	O								A	R		R	

Glossary of Terms

ADT: Admission, Discharge, and Transfer
Admission, Discharge, and Transfer systems are software systems used by healthcare facilities to track patients from arrival through to departure.

AHS: Allscripts
Leading provider of point-of-care decision support solutions for physicians.

CBA: Cost/Benefit Analysis
A technique designed to determine the feasibility of a project or plan by quantifying its costs and benefits.

CIS: Clinical Information System

CPOE: Computerized Provider Order Entry

CPR: Computer-based Patient Record (See EMR, EHR)

CSF: Critical Success Factors
Critical success factors are those objectives, tactics, and operational activities that define what the organization identifies as necessary to its success.

DUR: Drug Utilization Review
Study of drug prescriptions to evaluate a medication's usage and cost-effectiveness; may also be used to analyze treatment choices by individual practitioners, to suggest alternative medications, or to update an organization's drug formulary.

eHealth: Narrowly, the use of Web-based technologies to help consumers more actively participate as fully empowered partners in the health care team. More broadly, the organized transmission of medical information via Web-based or wireless technologies.

EMessaging and eVisits: Secure electronic messaging that enables patients, physicians, and other members of the health care team to communicate about certain types of health issues.

EMR: Electronic Medical Record: Electronic medical record. Also referred to as CPR, computerized patient record or PHR, patient health record, it includes the medical chart, health history, insurance information, lab results, drug allergies, etc.

EHR: Electronic Health Record. A fully evolved EMR, which extends care beyond the four walls of the doctor's office to include eHealth and other remote health transactions.

FTE: Full Time Equivalent: Full Time Equivalent (Employee) is an employee who works 40 hours per week, 52 weeks each year.

HIPAA: Health Insurance Portability and Accountability Act
Refers to the Health Insurance Portability and Accountability Act of 1996.

IDDUINEM: An acronym that stands for "If doctors don't use it, nothing else matters."

IDN: Integrated Delivery Network. A unified system of healthcare provision for its members including physician, hospital and ambulatory care services by contracting with several provider sites and health plans

IM: Instant Messaging. The ability to easily see whether a chosen friend or co-worker is connected to the Internet and, if they are, to exchange messages with them.

iPaq: Version of a PDA produced by Hewlett Packard

IS: Information Services. Common name for the organizational department that is responsible for data processing and information systems.

IT: Information Technology. IT is a term that encompasses all forms of technology used to create, store, exchange, and use information in its various forms.

KPI: Key Performance Indicator. A measure designed to track an identified critical performance variable over time.

LHII: Local Health Information Infrastructure

MOA: Medical Office Assistant

NIC: Network Interface Card. A card that is installed in a computer, enabling it to connect to a network.

NHII: National Health Information Infrastructure. An initiative set forth to improve the effectiveness, efficiency and overall quality of health and health care in the United States.

ROI: Return on investment. A measure of the revenue or savings a business will realize from any given undertaking.

PACS: Picture Archiving and Communication System. Electronic system used to exchange X-rays, CT scans, ultrasound and other medical images over a network.

PDA: Personal Digital Assistant. PDA is a term for any small, mobile hand-held device that provides computing and information storage. They are often used for keeping schedule calendars and address book information.

PCP: Primary Care Provider

PHR: Portable Health Record or Personal Health Record

PM: Project Manager. The individual responsible for managing a project.

PMS: Practice Management System

QA: Quality Assurance. The process of assuring that a product or service meets its specified requirements.

SAN: Storage Area Network. High-speed network that connects different kinds of data storage devices with associated data servers.

SIG: Prescription disbursement. This Latin term, which is frequently used in medicine and pharmacy, means "label" or "let it be imprinted."

TAT: Turn Around Time. The time it takes for an item to be processed.

WiFi: Wireless Fidelity (IEEE 802.11b wireless networking).

Author Biographies

Jed Batchelder has helped dozens of healthcare organizations implement Electronic Health Records (EHR) and has managed large upgrade projects with a number of organizations. Jed, who has also worked as a network support technician for a telecommunications consulting firm, holds a B.S. in computer science.

Bruce Buerger has more than a decade's worth of experience in information technology, including implementing and supporting healthcare systems as a Project Manager. A former adjunct professor at the Milwaukee School of Engineering, Bruce also previously worked as a managing consultant and mobile technology lead with a national IT consulting firm. In addition to his healthcare implementation experience, Bruce has participated in several large enterprise efforts in other industries.

Jason Carmichael has worked on numerous EHR implementations, including serving as Project Manager. Jason has also served as a software consultant, installation consultant, and interface analyst. He holds a BS in management information systems.

Michael Cassarino, an implementation Project Manager, has worked for several software development companies and for IBM. Michael is a Microsoft Certified Systems Engineer, and he holds an MBA in technology management.

Simon Curtis has led and contributed to more than twenty successful EHR implementations at academic medical centers, independent multi-specialty organizations, hospitals, IDNs, and specialty provider groups. A Project Manager since 2000, Simon has more than seven years of wide-ranging healthcare experience.

Peter Geerlofs, M.D., is the Chief Medical Officer of Allscripts. Dr. Geerlofs is the founder of Medifor, a medical software company, as well as a board-certified family physician, former county health officer, and founder of Port

Townsend Family Physicians, Inc. Since the early 1980s, Dr. Geerlofs has lectured and written widely on the use of computers in clinical medicine. He serves on the Steering Group of the Markle Foundation's "Connecting for Health Initiative," a public-private collaborative designed to address the challenges of mobilizing information to improve quality, conduct timely research, empower patients to become full participants in their care, and bolster the public health infrastructure.

Cristina Godwin brings more than nine years of healthcare experience to her role as a Project Manager. Cristina also has worked as a private HIT consultant, specializing in process re-engineering and improvement, and strategy and planning for hospitals and managed care companies. Cristina holds an MBA with a concentration in finance and healthcare services.

Brian Krupski has more than twelve years of wide-ranging healthcare software experience with clinical information systems for ambulatory medical records, radiology imaging and information systems. Brian's experience has enabled him to bring value to clients through his roles in software development, solution implementations, support services and process excellence. Brian was principle architect of Allscripts' EHR implementation methodology, based on Six Sigma principles, which the company launched in January 2004.

Maryse Laforce spent fourteen years at IDX Systems Corporation's Internet subsidiary, ChannelHealth, working in the Installation and Customer Service departments within the Enterprise Systems and Radiology Divisions. At Allscripts, Maryse is responsible for all customer implementation and service activities, and has worked with many other customers in a consultative role assisting with their charge implementations. Maryse holds a B.S. in computer science.

Laurie McGraw spent thirteen years at IDX Systems Corporation's Internet subsidiary, ChannelHealth, focusing on clinical automation in various roles running implementations, development and service groups. Today, Laurie is responsible for Allscripts' TouchWorks business unit. Laurie recently served on the 2004 Board of Examiners for the Baldrige National Quality Program.

Dan Michelson, Allscripts' Chief Marketing Officer, drives the company's 'go-to-market' strategy. Dan has served in leadership roles related to strategic planning, product management, marketing and sales for Baxter Healthcare, a leading medical supply company, and AstraZeneca, one the world's largest pharmaceutical companies. Additionally, he spent a number of years providing strategy and process redesign consulting services to many of the leading hospitals and integrated delivery networks in the U.S. In all roles in his career, his primary focus has been on driving meaningful change to improve healthcare. Dan holds a B.S. in finance and an M.B.A. in marketing and management.

Matt Nice has served in a variety of roles in healthcare information technology, most recently as a Project Manager. Matt previously worked for CCC Information Services, where he managed the Northern California region.

Bonnie Schirato drives Allscripts' internal and external education programs as Vice President of Human Resources. Bonnie spent eleven years in sporting goods retail, including positions in store operations, multi-unit field management, recruiting, corporate and field training and education, and overall employee relations. Bonnie holds a B.A. in English.

Andrew Sears has contributed to a number of EHR implementations. Andrew holds a B.A. in business administration with a concentration in MIS.

Jerry Seufert is the founder of the management consulting firm Fresh Air. Jerry has led clinical systems projects since the 1970's, and has particular expertise in implementation process, achieving high doctor utilization, and managing software-enabled operations transformation. His unique understanding of how doctors engage—and don't engage—with software has contributed to many successful implementations.

Glen E. Tullman is Chief Executive Officer of Allscripts. Glen was formerly Chief Executive Officer of Enterprise Systems, Inc., a publicly traded healthcare information services company providing resource management solutions to large integrated healthcare networks. Prior to that, Glen was President and Chief Operating Officer of CCC Information Services Group, Inc., a computer software company servicing the insurance industry. He has worked for the Executive Office of the President in Washington, D.C., and has also served as a guest lecturer at the Harvard School of Business and the Wharton School of Business. As a social anthropologist trained at St. Anthony's College, Oxford University, Glen's interest in human behavior guides Allscripts' efforts to help healthcare professionals manage the change from traditional processes to technologically enhanced workflows.

Editor's Biography

Todd Stein is a former Sacramento Bee reporter and an award-winning free-lance writer and editor whose work has appeared in numerous national publications. Between 2000 and 2003, Todd wrote and produced HIMSS Newsbreak, a weekly Internet broadcast program on healthcare technology for the members of the Healthcare Information and Management Systems Society. Today, he continues to write about HIT for several industry publications. He holds a BA in journalism.